PE____

By

Pamela V Johnson DNP, MSN - APRN, FNP-BC

@

ConsultIdaNP

Publisher: ConsultIdaNP

https://www.consultidanp.com

ISBN: 978-1-7325867-0-3 eBook
ISBN: 978-1-7325867-1-0 paperback

Dedication

PEEPED is dedicated to people who dare to 'become' in spite of circumstances. Abuse, bullying, domestic and intimate partner violence are acquired and learned behaviors. Abusive, bullying, and violent behaviors are unhealthy means of expressing emotions. These behaviors can and do spill into adulthood. Abusing and bullying are never warranted. There are healthier ways to express how you feel and to ask for what you want. Healthy relationships include abilities to share in mutual understandings, as well as respectful disagreements.

Glimpse

Prelude

What happened in the past isn't always relevant to the future. Living Beyond Survival: Laughing, Loving, Sharing...*Life!*, was a prelude, partial accounting, relevant to outcomes. A reminder that the saying, "We cannot fight what we cannot see" is Erroneous! Wars are won against the unknown every moment of each day.

1 Corinthians 4:5 "Therefore judge nothing before the time, until the Lord come, who both will bring to light the hidden things of darkness, and will make manifest the counsels of the hearts; and then shall every man have praise of God (VerseWise Bible, KJV)."

Chapter I

The Lone Twig

Outside, along the wall, underneath the balcony of this fourth floor hotel room is one lone twig; resembling a branch as though on a tree. This lone twig is healthy, green in color and covered with multiple leaves.

Unique in its place, out of character, this lone twig, a thin piece of a branch from a tree has majestically survived and thrived. At this height, its' roots invisible, appear to have grown up, and through concrete and mortar. A single thin twig reaching up and out...it faces west as the sun rises in the east. *Amazing*!

If this twig could answer, I would ask, "Where are you anchored? To what are your roots attached?" And I would say to this lone twig, "Great JOB! Whatever birthed you, has shared in life with you, sustained you, is simply...*GOOD*." This lone twig shown as a patch of nature in concrete, is a reminder of how simple life really can be - *Is*! Just like this lone twig, substance isn't taken...substance is given...*shared*.

Although support structures of this lone twig are not visible, the stalk to which leaves cling, and the environmental elements that sustain its' life are a mystery. Erect, not adhered to structures of the building; green, surviving. No other species of its kind are in site. Are our lives like this lone twig? Planted, nurtured, and brought forth to thrive?

Ezekiel 17: 5 – 6, "He took also of the seed of the land and planted it in a fruitful field; he placed it by great waters and set it as a willow tree. And it grew and became a spreading vine of low stature, whose branches turned towards him, and the roots thereof were under him; so it became a vine and brought forth branches, and shot forth sprigs."

Mini Moments are memorable times in our lives that make a difference. Good, bad, or indifferent...we all have memories of random events important to who we have become. If having a second chance meant correcting something of the past, something that would make things as you believe they should be, where would you begin? If your list is long, or unimaginable, you should have done it right the first time. A person can spend countless hours making efforts to change yesterday. Is it worth it? What are a few of your 'Mini Moments'?

Mini Moment #1: Reflect: What, if anything, would you change?

_____

_____

_____

_____

_____

_____

Have you tried to change?

_____

_____

_____

_____

_____

_____

_____

Mimi Moment #2: Reflect: What, if anything,
would you change?

_____

_____

_____

_____

_____

_____

_____

Have you tried to change?

_____

_____

_____

_____

_____

_____

_____

_____

_____

Chapter II

A Beginning...

Late night phone calls...stolen moments to share thoughts. Whispers across air waves...communication. Care...free...exchanges of friendship, affection, joy. Consensual, without lust. Not lust of consciousness or flesh. Building relations..."friendships"...pure innocence, shared. Who knows details of what is not shared?

Friendships between people with likes, similar ideas...; Differences...in appearance, aptitude, various religious preferences, etc... Late night calls, text messages, exchanges of communication...being. Exchanges of communication do not define relationships. Is there a relationship? Or is exchange of communication essential in being? Being yourself? Being with another? Perception of self? Perceptions of others? Is one's ability to communicate important to understanding who you are becoming, who you have become?

Right now, at this moment, can you see yourself? Look at the space in front of you: I sit in a room. An empty room. An empty room with one chair. A chair with tripod legs, a swivel base and no back. There is no door to this room. No way out and no way in. Yet I am not alone. No other persons are capable of sharing space within this room. There is one window.

Within this room there is life: particles exchanged between flesh and the environment. There are pastel colors on the walls, a few pictures of things once important. Memories of what was; places visited, people important…with whom lifes' paths have crossed. A glimpse, a stare, passive omissions like thieves passing in the dark. Perceptions that can be mistaken, misunderstood, overlooked, or acknowledged. Unspoken communications exchanged.

1 Corinthians 13: 11 "When I was a child, I spoke as a child, I understood as a child, I thought as a child; but when I became a man, I put away childish things."

Chapter III

Begin...Then, what?!

Research that describes psychology of relationships is insurmountable. So much, that people might forget to use common sense. One's perceptions interacting with another is important to self and the other. If or how we share our perceptions and expectations (if any) with others can be daunting.

Age appropriate social skills ... *WHAT?!* Does a six month old infant respond to familiar faces and attitudes of their parents the same as when that toddler is 16 months of age? They shouldn't, but might.

Does a 5 year old child develop friendships the same as at age the age of 10? Maybe.

Do we expect a 16 year old to have social skills of a 26 year old? Many do...!

At the age of 56, do we expect to have the same features, personality and social skills as at the age of 30? Some do...!

Thus, personality disorders develop that are not diagnosed until something happens.

Dependent children can grow into immature, needy adolescent adults. Become clingy, emotionally needy, never feeling fulfilled, lacking verification of self-identity. Identify is essential to becoming and feeling nurtured.

Or, the sixteen-month-old infant matures, learns to socialize with other infants, toddlers, then children, and displays appropriate behaviors with the right people in the right places for the right reasons..., then becomes a healthy adult ... with hidden agendas.

Perhaps the five-year-old is secretly introduced to "child's play" - intimate touch, by a 10-year-old. Untold secrets, reassurance of false security says, "Someone will take care of me, if I comply." There goes the self-esteem; values of self vs worth.

Then there is the sixteen-year-old, who at the age of twenty-six is still seeking an "identity." Having not completed any tasks or accomplished something of meaning that could have helped (oneself) answer the question, "Who am I?" This person's behavior might resemble that of a child.

———

Last, but not least, is a fifty-six-year-old fearful of embracing who they have become. Beginnings, influences, do not have to determine who we become. Nor should who we are, or who we are becoming adversely affect the lives of others.

As children, like begets like. As adults, friendships are (should be) complementary relationships, with mutual purposes. What happens when we engage others in friendship without abilities to communicate openly and honestly?

Ability to accept rejection from another is just as import as rejecting another. Think back to infancy; were you emotionally or physically needy as a child? If you do not recall, ask someone who remembers.

Do you require validation from another in order to complete tasks, make decisions, or to feel complete? Are you capable of making decisions with another? ... For another?

Test yourself. Dine alone in public, sit through a movie alone, go to your favorite place alone. Let yourself feel, be present with you!

Journal your thoughts and feelings of whatever event you chose to complete alone. If you are not comfortable writing your thoughts and feelings on paper, allow yourself time to internalize your feelings - in real time. Enjoy the moment, this is your mini moment. Your life is *YOUR* journey.

Some people prefer group dynamics, crowds, and developing many friendships. Some people prefer to be alone or in small groups.

There are people who will accept your becoming, as well as who you are. Some people prefer accepting and respecting others for who they have become without naming relationships (e.g., friends, lovers, sibling, etc.). Socialization is a learned process.

Do not expect from another what you give. Share with expectation that gifts shared with another are gifts received. Gifts of gratitude: like smiles instead of frowns, praise instead of constant critiques; a helping hand, not a handout.

Some people may not receive what is given in context of a "gift." Others may not be capable of sharing of themselves (emotions, time, presence,

… etc.). The same gift shared between different people, in the same situation, may not be perceived with the same meaning. In other words, just because we share the same gifts with others does not mean the other with whom words, prayers, time, a glance, a hug, less or more intimate gestures used to communicate resonate a clear message. If in doubt…don't. Once done, we cannot undo an action nor verbiage. We can be authentic, disagreeable, honest, caring, and present…as self.

Irregardless of how we began, who we have become is who we are NOW! Allowing others' perceptions of who they need you to be is not natural.

An immature child can become an emotionally dependent high functioning executive unable to function without controlling behaviors of another. For example, their spouse must be as envisioned, the children must behave as expected, or plans at work must be goal directed. Unspoken words and actions, like micromanaging household finances as a means of control can lead to abnormal interactions with others. These behaviors are generally shown in what is known as abuse, bullying, domestic or intimate partner violence.

Abuse, bullying, domestic and intimate partner violence are not limited to age, gender, race, ethnicity, nor socioeconomic status. There are no borders - until behaviors associated with abuse, bullying, domestic or intimate partner violence are exposed.

Know thy self! De-escalate behaviors associated with abuse, bullying, domestic and intimate partner violence by understanding that an abuser or bully are not in control. Abusers and bullies have unmet needs; they need to be in control. Abusers and bullies lack control of something intimate, personal, or unfulfilled.

People who are abusive or bullies may not realize their behaviors are not normal. Aggression is a means of expressing anger. Abusers and bullies need and will usually *not* seek help to control themselves (***their behavior***).

Similar to a hunter rejoicing after capture of the hunted, an abuser or bully internalizes their feelings and are fulfilled having demeaned another. *Know thyself!* Learn to recognize potential symptoms of abusive and bullying behaviors.

Wisdom of Solomon 19:18 (VerseWise) "For the elements were changed in themselves by a kind of harmony, like as in a psaltery notes change the name of the tune, and yet as always sounds; which may well be perceived by the sight of the things that have been done."

Chapter IV

Enter into Relationships

Experts write about four common stages in "Cycles of Abuse." Calm, tension building, eruption of an event (physical, psychological, verbal), and reconciliation (making up). There is no expected order to the cycles of abuse. Abuse, bullying, domestic and intimate partner violence is about "control" or "lack of control."

During the calm phase of a relationship, everything seems okay. Perhaps you have just entered into a friendship or have been committed for years. Your expectations as individuals will differ. How people chose to express themselves is important in any relationship. Characteristics of the 'Calm phase' are described as a time when no abuse is taking place and the relationship seems to be going well.

It is possible to dismiss abuse and bullying given labels placed on relationships (e.g., lovers, friends, siblings, parents, etc.). Nor are you expected to know what someone expects, without clarifying their expectations, if expectations exist.

People meet and form relationships. Relationships aren't always viewed by each person involved, in the same manner. Relationships affect many, not just a few.

Mini Moment:

A mutual friend arranges a conversation. They share likes through internet and phone conversations over time. One has siblings. The other is an only child.

One is graduating college while working part time. The other owns a small business and will enter college in the fall. Eventually, they agree to meet, face to face.

Interactive social media has done justice for one, but not for the other. Their personalities sync. Time spent over lunch has been delightful.

Through mutual agreement, they enjoy several outings, laughing and sharing stories. They go bowling, play tennis, swim within a Community Center's pool.

One day they casually meet while roaming through an outlet mall. The college student is with a friend. The two spot one another as they approach. They wave from across the aisle, share smiles, and continue in opposite directions. Two days later while talking over the phone, they agree to meet for coffee.

It's early, 6 pm on a Friday evening. The Student sits thinking, 'I'll have a seltzer with a hint of lemon and review today's biology notes while waiting. My new friend is 20 minutes late.' A text message arrives.

Friend: "Run'g bhnd, OTW." After two drinks, the Student is accompanied.

Student: "Hi, how was your day?"

Friend: "Busy, but productive."

Student: "Tell me more about your small business. It is exiting to talk with someone under the age of 20 that owns a business."

Friend: "My mom sold beauty products from home when we were young. She taught us how to do business as way to earn our own money when my brother and I were about 17 and 18. My brother and I joined mom in partnership and work as time permits to ensure internet orders are filled, distributions are complete, and customer reviews are favorable. Was that your brother with you in the mall?"

Student: "No." As she smiles and glances across the table at her new friend.

Friend: "Tell me about college life. I begin taking classes part time this fall."

Student: "Oh. Where?"

Friend: "At Inner City Junior College."

Student: "What is your area of interest, business?"

Friend: "Sort of. Health Sciences and Art."

Student: "I should be ready to begin nursing core courses this fall. The University requires prerequisites be complete before permitting entry into courses that involve interaction with the public."

Friend: "So, you are a nursing student?"
Student "Yes."

Friend: "And your friend? Is he a nursing student too?"

Student: "No." No explanations are offered. "How do health sciences and art relate to business?"

Friend: "Health sciences as well as study of the arts, offer knowledge that can be used as I build a career. Creating a path that includes happiness as I earn money is important to who I will become. Business includes processes implemented as one strategizes to use knowledge through transition of power while earning a living."

The story continues and events lead to "Tension Building." Days, weeks, then a month later one calls the other.

Friend: "Hi. How are you?"

Student: "Hi. Well, thank you?"

Friend: "I have been thinking about you, no…us. When are you free to get together this or next week?"

Student: "I'm not sure. What were you thinking we should do?"

Friend: "I'm not sure. I miss talking with you."

Student: "Okay. Would you like to join me for a swim at the Community Center tomorrow afternoon?"

Friend: "No. Tomorrow isn't a good day. How about Thursday afternoon, around 5 o'clock?"

Student: "I swim three or more days a week. I'm at the Community Center on Monday's and Thursday's. Other days, I swim closer to home, early mornings, before class."

Friend: "Where do you live?"

Student: "In an apartment off campus. I swim between 6 and 7 in the morning and do not invite anyone to my home that early."

Friend: "Tell me more about your place."

Student: "Meet me at the Community Center Thursday or Monday afternoon. I'm usually in the pool by 5 or 5:30 p.m."

Friend (*thinking*): 'What just happened? No information on him - the friend. No contact in a month. I thought we were becoming friends. The guy from the mall must be significant. Maybe there is no interest in an us. It seemed we were growing closer.'

———

Two days pass. It's Thursday and a male friend from school has decided to share a lane and swim laps this evening with the student and her friend. Student (*thinking*): 'My friend might join us. Three or four people can share one lane.'

The Friend arrives.

Student "Hi. We have been in the water about thirty minutes. Join us, we swim in circles to avoid bumping into one another. I usually swim fifty laps; Twenty-five in each direction."

Friend (*unspoken*): 'Whow! The boyfriend is swimming with us! This is not what I expected. The circle of two had increased to three. She expects three people to swim laps freestyle in one lane.'

The school mate, male friend, leaves after completing 35 laps. A while later, the college student completes fifty laps and gets out of the pool. The new friend swims two more laps, then comes onto the deck.

Friend: "Thanks, I needed to exercise. I didn't realize how much stress one can relieve exercising. And you do this a few days a week?"

25

Student: "Yeah. Studying requires concentration. I too, work as a nursing assistant three to four days a week to pay tuition."

Friend: "Really? You didn't tell me that? How can you work and attend classes full time?"

Student: "I exercise and prioritize responsibilities."

Friend: "So, are you and that guy involved?"

Student "Yes."

Friend: "So, why didn't you tell me you're involved?"

Student: "Thou assumes too much. What do you mean by 'involved'?"

Friend: "We haven't talked much over the past month and today he is here when I arrive. What gives? Why didn't you tell me he would be joining us? It would have been nice to know we would not be alone."

Tension continues to build with our new friend. Our working student feels no pressure. The Student smiles at the Friend and extends an invitation to go for coffee.

Friend: "What will you have - coffee, a latte, a frappuccino?"

Student: "No, I will buy my own coffee. Thanks."

Friend: "Okay." Each purchases a beverage, then they sit adjacent to one another sharing small talk.

Friend: "So, I tell you I miss talking to you and you invite someone to join us during a swim?"

Student: "It sounds as though his presence upset you."

Friend: "I love your hair and your smile and the way I feel after talking to you. I thought we were building a relationship."

Student: "We are. But to me, conversations and sharing in activities of interest are ways to build friendships. I have more friends than time."

Friend: "I tell you things that I don't share with anyone. And you dismiss me as though our friendship is common! I had hoped we could spend more time together, as a couple."

Student: "Your friendship is important to me. But between school and work, there is little time to consider entering a serious or intimate relationship. If I have in any way made you believe differently, please accept an apology."

Friend: "How could you have not known?"

Student: "We seem to have different views on the subject of relationships. Just as we differ on what it means to be involved. I consider us to be friends and we are involved, but for me there is no interest in romance; emotional or physical. Let's talk about this later, I have to work tonight." She stands to leave, "If you are interested in exercising with a friend, I'll be in the pool Monday and Thursday evenings after 5."

The Friend thinks: 'Meet her for a swim, really? I'll follow to see where she works. What kind of work can she do tonight? *Humm....*' She follows her to someone's home. 'I knew it! She's meeting him! Why won't she just tell me that he's her boyfriend?'

The next day, the Friend phones: "Hi."

Student: "Hi."

Friend: "I'm sorry I upset you yesterday. I really enjoy talking and being with you. Maybe we should slow down and give one another space? What do you think?"

Student: "Okay."

Monday afternoon. They arrive at the pool different times. The friend watched as the Student entered the water, then got into a different lane and began swimming laps. Thirty minutes pass, then an hour. 'She is still swimming! I will swim a few more laps then wait for her in the locker room.'

The Friend gets out of the pool and begins searching for the Student: 'Where is she? She isn't in the water. She isn't on the deck. She isn't in the locker room. Maybe she is in the shower? Could she have left for work? I don't know where she lives. I will text her.' Text: "Hi, wh'r R U?"

The Student returns a text: "Hm"

Friend texts "Oh. Mst uv mis U @the pool."

Student text: "Next time."

The next day, the Friend texts the student: "Gd Mrng. Do U hv plns Sat?"

An hour later, the student returns a text: "Yes."

Friend's text: "I hv a prob & rlly Nd a frnd. Meet at coffee shop Sat mrng?"

Student text "No gd. Sun after 3?"

Friend text "K."

Sunday afternoon at the coffee shop the Friend arrives early: 'I have been waiting 30 minutes! Where is she?!' Enter the working college Student: "Hi."

Friend: "Thanks for coming. Can I get you a coffee?"

Student: "No thanks, I'm good. What's going on?"

Friend: "I've been thinking about us. I offended you like a jealous partner last week. Please forgive me. It's been sometime since my last relationship and dating feels new to me."

Student: "We have to stop talking and meeting."

Friend: "Why?"

Student: "You assume I want an intimate partnership with you. I appreciate our conversations, and time shared with people with whom I have things in common. But I am not interested in being intimate with anyone. So, perhaps we should not talk, text or meet again. I wish you well, sincerely."

Friend: "Wait! Your brother and I have planned a surprise outing this week. Aren't you coming with him to the opera Friday evening?"

Student: "What brother? Exactly, what did you say?"

Friend: "I told him we have become very close friends, and asked what I might do to strengthen our relationship? He told me you like Theater, including the Opera, so I decided to invite you and him, along with his friend - out.

I purchased four tickets and gave your brother three. I plan to meet you in the Mezzanine's balcony at 6:30 pm. The show begins at 7 o'clock."

Student: "How did you meet my brother?"

Friend: "We passed in the mall."

Student: "But, I haven't introduced you to my brother, so what made you think some guy from the mall is MY BROTHER?!"

Friend: "Hon, we have been together a long time. I don't remember who found whom. I don't remember if he called me or I called him."

Student: "Why would my brother call you?"

Friend: "We hang out."

LATER...

The Student talking to a colleague: "Hello 'Dear Brother'. I have a new friend with whom you have become too talkative. Do you have Opera tickets?"

Colleague: "Yes, why?"

Student: "Did you promise to accompany me and one of your friends to the Opera this Friday evening?"

Colleague: "I planned to ask you to join us, why?"

Student: "Did you ask why this person wants to surprise me? How long have you known this person and how did you meet?"

Colleague: "We met at a coffee shop. She thought we were lovers. But, I told her that we are brother and sister. Then she invited us to the Opera. What is the big deal?"

Student 'Okay' she thinks, 'So, this girl believes she knows more about me than I have shared. And my *brother* is her muse.'

Student sends a text to the Friend: "Se U Fri nite?"

Friends returned text "K. dnr after?"

They met in the lobby of the Theater:

Student (*thinking*): 'My colleague and cousin are by my side. She hugged me, ran her hand along my arm, then gently touched the back of my hand.'

Friend: "Thanks for accepting my invitation."

After the show ... Friend: "That was magnificent! There is an Italian restaurant around the corner. Reservations aren't required."

Student: "Okay. Let me have a few moments with my colleague and cousin."

The friend thinks: 'Colleague? Cousin?'

Student: "Excuse us please. I will meet you outside in a few minutes."

Friend (*to herself*): 'What, a colleague? Does she expect me to believe he is a colleague? I have waited six months too long. Tonight we confirm our relationship as partners.'

A waiter approached their table: "How may I serve you?"

Student: "I'll have seltzer with a splash of lemon juice."

Waiter: "Would you like to have an appetizer?"

Student: "No."

Waiter: "And you, Mam?" referring to the Friend. "Please, bring us a bottle of Cabernet. We will share a mini anchovy pizza with extra white cheddar as an appetizer." The waiter, smiles, nods at each of them, then leaves.

Student: "I have tried to be nice to you. There is no *WE*! There is me and you. We are NOT a couple. I have no interest and will not pretend to be interested in sharing my personal self with you. (*She smiles*) We, will never happened!"

Friend: "Oh, but you will. As evidenced by our meeting this evening. We are here, now. We have been together for a long time. Over six months. I knew when we met, you were interested. We girls have to stick together. Don't worry. No one will know, yet. Let's move on, shall we?"

The Student is silently enraged. She contemplates walking out, but that would be rude. This is embarrassing. What else has she done to learn about my life? (*Speaking*) "Dinner was, interesting. I have school, then work this week. Please, do not contact me again." She stands, turns to leave and says, "This moment was to say good-bye, so long," then walks away. Once out the door and in her car, her phone pings. A picture of the two of them, appearing to embrace has been posted on a social media site. It reads, "Together at last." *What?!*

The Student receives a text message from the Friend: "U R mine. Thks for a grt nite. See U shrtly √."

At this point, the Student is seeing RED! 'I have been violated, bullied, and abused! How is she stalking me? She is obsessed! I cannot control her behavior, but I can reinforce a NO GO of this presumed "partnership!" '

Break!

Decisions to reconcile differences (or to make up) should be mutual. Input from each person involved is important. You are your best friend. Once you begin to like and accept who you are, as well as who you are becoming, or who you have become, what has been, what was - just is.

Abusers and bullies may not accept that their behaviors are "abnormal." Remember, abuse, bullying, domestic and intimate partner violence are not limited to race, sex, age, or nationality.

People with unmet needs can and will lash out using silence, can become combative, might isolate their prey by befriending and manipulating the environment or people surrounding their intended victim.

Proverbs 3:27 "Withhold not good from them to whom it is due, when it is in the power of thine hand to do it." KJV

STOP!!

Reflect on the story in the "mini moment" above. Can you relate behaviors and characteristics to yourself, or to someone you know? Are you reminded of a similar situation? What, if anything, from this story is important to you?

_____

_____

_____

_____

_____

_____

_____

_____

_____

_____

Why?_____

_____

_____

_____

_____

_____

_____

_____

_____

_____

_____

_____

_____

_____

_____

Chapter V

FORWARD...

There is an old saying, "Association brings about assimilation." Meaning, people become like those with whom they associate. Maybe, but not necessarily.

Similarly, there is another cliché, "People become products of their environment." That too, is debatable. What we learn, is not what we 'know.' There are people who do not realize how mutilated their self-esteem really – IS!

Mini Moment...

A father says, "Boy, you will never be nothin'! You are just like your lazy momma. That's why I left her. Do you know why I'm raising you instead of your momma? I'm a man! And a boy needs a man. A woman cannot raise a boy to be a man. Women can only be laid or give birth to a boy."

At the age of 6, Micky hears his father's words and those words sting worse than the bite of a hornet! He loves them; both parents. But, this child only knows how to show his emotions.

41

Micky walks away from his dad with his head hanging down, his eyes focused on the ground in front of him, tears welting in his eyes, shoulders slumped. What has he done wrong? How can he make his father proud? Micky tries to see himself through his father's eyes. Micky believes his father expects him to be strong, determined, and a hard worker. But, something is missing. There is an emptiness that cannot be explained. Micky misses his mother and does not have female friends.

Micky didn't understand why his father hit his mom. Memories of his parent's relationship are vague. That morning she left for work began like any other day. They had breakfast as a family, Micky got into the car with his mom and on the way to school she spoke in a whisper, "I love you. Don't ever forget that. What happens between me and your dad doesn't have anything to do with you. One day, you will understand."

At the age of 4, Micky hears, but does not understand. He internalizes his feelings, not sure of how to behave, unable to say how he feels.

———

42

Emotions can lead to "actions in motion." Too often, people act out their feelings. But, feelings aren't always made clear though actions. People's opinions (perceptions) of another aren't always accurate. Lack of communication can lead to misinterpretation of behaviors (aka: emotions = actions in motion).

Over the years, Micky hasn't made many friends. He isn't allowed to play outside until his dad comes home from work. His dad takes Micky to school at 7:30 each morning. Micky walks home alone after school. He has been taught not to speak to strangers, and to never bring anyone into the house.

His after-school routine is the same: take off your shoes at the door, make sure your bedroom is clean, then clean the kitchen. It's okay to watch television or to play video games but complete your homework before dinner. His dad is usually home before 6 pm and they have dinner together between 7 and 7:30 pm.

Micky's dad Jack is an executive at a bank downtown. Some weekends, Jack makes time to take Micky fishing or hunting. Jack's job requires him to travel at least one weekend a month. When Jack travels, Micky stays home alone or one of Jack's lady friends sleeps over.

Jack seems to have a lot a 'lady friends.' One of Jack's friends, Ms. TK, allows Micky to sleep with her in Jack's bed when Jack is away. Late night talks, watching television in bed helps Micky fall asleep. Atmosphere in the house is quiet and serene when Jack is away.

Micky feels he is too old to sleep alongside his father's friend, but TK coos him like a mother providing security or safety to her child.

Silently, Micky questions what their relationship would have been like had his mother been around? She is missed. Micky can't talk with his father about his interest in girls. Talking with TK is out of the question. She might be one of his father's girlfriends, but she is not considered Micky's friend or mother.

At the age of eleven, Micky's dad is asked by a neighbor if Micky can play intermural football. Some weekends, Micky watches football on television. He has learned "the game" of football is about running, touching and hitting another.

Coaches teach Micky how to be 'goal directed and disciplined.' The primary goal in football is to WIN! Team members compliment Micky saying he is smart, articulate, and a leader that follows through. All the guys seem to like Micky, but his pinned-up anger has begun to present through aggressive behaviors.

The phone rings, it's Micky's dad. "I need you to come straight home after school this evening."

Micky: "Okay, What about Coach?"

Dad: "I'll call him."

As Micky approaches home, he notices two police cars in the driveway. What has happened? Two police officers are outside, one tires to prevent Micky from entering the house, but Micky spots his dad standing in the kitchen and runs towards him. Micky can see a woman sitting with her back to them, talking to a third police officer. The woman's hair is shoulder length, brown, and curly. That voice, he recognizes her voice. "Mom?"

She stands with her back to Micky and walks away, towards another room, "Don't let him see me like this. He can't see me like this."

"Dad, what's going on? What happened? What have you done?!" Micky shouts.

"Micky, not now! Take this up with me later." His dad walked away as Micky was escorted outside to a sit in a squad car. Sitting in the back seat, Micky can see one of the police officers standing in the yard with his dad. He hears portions of their conversation but doesn't understand why his mother came back. How could his father hate her? Why would Micky's dad want her "locked up?"

Micky is still sitting in the back seat of a police car when their eyes connect. The woman is accompanied by an Officer to a second police car. "That woman doesn't look like my mom." The woman is fat, her face is swollen, one eye has a large black and blue circle, there are dark spots on her face and neck. The collar of her shirt is torn, and her hair is disheveled. Tears fill Micky's eyes as he remembers the last time he saw his mother. He bangs on the window with questions, "This can't be her! Who is she? Why can't I talk to her?"

His dad opens the door to the car and barks at Micky to "get out of the car." Jack grabs Micky's arm and escorts him inside the house, an Officer follows. Then, Jack leaves Micky and returns outside.

Micky walks through the kitchen, into the living room, then towards his bedroom. He sees a broken chair laying on the floor, and one of two glass tables is broken. A trail of blood leads from the bathroom, into his bedroom. Micky notices a picture of he and his mom sitting on his dresser. He thinks, 'I don't remember when this was taken. How old was I? What could I have done that made her leave? What happened between mom and dad?'

Later that evening, Micky's dad calls him to the dinner table. Micky tires to talk with his dad, "Dad, was that mom? Why was she here?"

Micky's questions are dismissed. "Not now, son! One day you will understand! Never let a woman make demands in your house, son. It's your house, you make the rules! Remember that!" Without hearing an explanation, Micky has no way of getting answers to his questions. His father is present, but distant. His mother has left, again.

At the age of 15, Micky meets Jane. Micky thinks Jane is beautiful. Micky has admired Jane for weeks. Jane's skin is a pretty peach pecan brown. Her hair glows with a hint of red mixed with brown. Curves of this 14-year-old's body evokes arousal of feelings that Micky is not able to explain. Something within Micky awakens at the site of Jane. 'Does she know I'm watching?' A few of Micky's friends interrupt his thoughts. "Micky, let's go. Practice begins in 15 minutes."

Micky is a 'good team member' and as a sophomore he plays several positions on the varsity football team. Playing the position of guard on the offensive line, Micky has learned to prevent opponents from moving through the line. And as a defensive tackle, Micky can transfer internal anger into aggression on the field by hitting. He learns to hit opponents, hard!

His father rarely comes to a game. When his dad shows up, he is usually late and smells of alcohol. His dad coaches from the sidelines, not realizing how embarrassed Micky feels hearing his voice. "That's my son! Come on, you can do better than that. Stop that son of a b..-.ch, *HIT HIM!*"

Increasingly, Micky's anger is provoked by thoughts of his father's behavior. Nothing Micky does is every good enough. Micky begins to redirect his anger and hits an opponent really hard! He hears a whistle and the clock stops. A member of the other team is shaken, examined and declared "Okay" then escorted off the field. Coach looks at Micky with concern, 'What just happened?'

Micky has not talked to friends nor the coach about his life at home. Memories of his mother have begun to fade, yet occasionally he reminisces about what might have been.

Life with his father is hard. At the age of 16, it has become harder to disguise his feelings.

Micky believes his friendship with Jane is solid, but he does not talk about his father or himself with friends. A few of his buddies' whisper and joke, saying Micky talks to girls like they are slaves.

Micky, "Jane, tell the girls good-bye, I need to talk with you a minute."

Jane, "I'll catch up with you later, Micky. After cheerleading practice."

Micky, "No, now! I have things to do after football practice and this can't wait."

Jane, "Okay…" She turns to her friends, "I'll meet you in the gym."

Micky grabs Jane's arms firmly and pulls her close. As they walk away from Jane's friends, he kisses her cheek to show affection. Then whispers, "When I call, you come."

They continue along a corridor that leads into an outdoor grassy area towards a large oak tree, then behind a gazebo. Micky thrusts Jane against the gazebo, pulls her close, and attempts to kiss her on the lips, but she pushes him away and says, "NO!"

_____

Micky is shocked and embarrassed at his behavior. There have been times, Micky felt compelled to caress Jane, but this was not one of those moments! "We have been friends for a long time. You haven't ever shown an interest in me like this. What gives?" Retorts Jane.

Micky hesitates, then says, "I'm sorry." Then runs off. Jane is left standing beside the gazebo, wondering what just happened. She is pissed, to say the least, and expects to get answers to her questions.

Micky has blocked all thoughts of having assaulted Jane. He turns internal anger into aggression and assumes his position among teammates running drills on the football field. Unexplained rage has Micky pumped. After practice, he showers, changes and tells his friends he has something to do.

Micky decides to take a different path home. If he walks through the park and turns on 17th street, he will see Jane's house. Maybe, he will see Jane and straighten things out.

As Micky approaches the corner of 16th Terrace and 17th street, he spots Jane standing beside a car, talking with a few girls. He begins to walk towards Jane; she sees him coming and walks in his direction. Calmly Jane says, "Hi, what was that about?"

"I don't know." Micky explains that lately he has been thinking of a lot of things. "I really like you. I wouldn't ever think of hurting you. I guess, I thought being close to you would calm these feelings. I am sorry I scared you."

"Scared me?" Jane stares at Micky, "You didn't scare me. You violated me! You can't be trusted. We have shared a lot of secrets, and NEVER have you talked about being angry. I believed we were friends."

Micky, "We are! I messed up. That should never have happened. It won't happen again. Can we start over? As friends?" He smiles towards Jane, who says, "I'll consider the offer" as she walks back towards her friends.

Micky is now age 17 and a senior in high school. He and Jane as friends have accompanied one another on dates; there is romance, but no sexual intimacy.

Jane plans to attend college out of state next year and Micky hasn't decided if he will remain in state or accept a scholastic offer from a school out of state.

Mike a new kid from across town has transferred into their high school. Micky is asked to mentor his new teammate. Mike is in the 10th grade and has never played football.

Mike lives within the same neighborhood as Micky. One afternoon, while walking home from school, Mike invites Micky to play basketball. Everyday, they pass a basketball court on their way home. Maybe they can get together one Saturday afternoon to play, shoot a few hoops.

Mike, "Hey Micky, I have to do a few things around the house with my dad this evening. Why don't you come over Saturday around 10 o'clock, so we can shoot hoops?"

Micky "Let me talk with my dad. It should be okay. I'll text when on the way."

Saturday morning, Micky shows up at Mike's house around 9:45. Mike's dad has decided to go to the park with the boys to play a few games of basketball. Micky and Mike play a round to 21. Micky wins the first round, then plays Mike's dad.

After a few games, Micky is invited to Mike's house for lunch. This is the first time Micky has felt comfortable, like he has a real friend. Nor has Micky ever visited anyone without his dad being present. His dad is usually intrusive. Teammates are not allowed to visit Micky at home and phone calls are usually screened. Away from school, Micky has never bonded with boys his age.

During lunch, Mike's dad offers the boys a beer. Micky is surprised, but he does not speak or look at Mike or his dad. Mike's father has never offered him alcohol. Mike knows that his dad becomes mean when drinking and his mother is out of town on business.

When Mike's dad drinks, sometimes he says or does things. Things that are

———

embarrassing. Things Mike hasn't told his mom or his buddies. Things that he must prevent others from knowing. He thinks, "If my dad drinks too much and touches Micky, I'll....! He wouldn't."

Mike silently texts Micky while hiding the phone under the table, "? Meet me before practice M'day? Dn't understand plays."

Micky feels his phone vibrate, he reads the message, looks up at Mike with a poker face and says, "Thanks for lunch. Gotta go." Micky finishes eating and leaves.

Monday morning Mike and Micky meet in the hall, "Hey, what was that message at lunch about?" Micky asked.

Mike nods and says, "Nothing, I could see you were ready to go." Micky doesn't believe Mike, nor does he make this an issue.

Micky will be 18 before graduating in June. He has begun to question his sexuality. He has gone out on dates with other girls who find him attractive, but he remains silently obsessed with Jane. He keeps up with where she goes, with whom, how often, and an app on his phone allows him to secretly track her whereabouts.

Micky gave Jane a clock shaped like a cheerleader for her 16th birthday. Unbeknown to Jane, there is a camera hidden behind the doll's eyes. Micky logs into his computer to access the doll and monitors Jane's actions within her bedroom.

Mike and Micky have become best friends. One day, they stop at the basketball court on the way home. Micky has noticed unexplained changes in Mike's behavior. "What's up with you?" Micky asked.

Mike, "What do you mean?"

Micky, "Something is different. It's like you are hiding something."

Mike, "Nothing. Everything is the same. The same schist, different day."

Micky, "Okay. You know what you say to me, stays with me."

As they prepare to leave the park, Mike asked Micky if he really meant what he said about keeping conversations private. Micky acknowledges with a smile and says, "yeah." Mike stops dribbling the basketball and says, "I would like to ask Mia to prom, but..."

"So, what's the big deal?" Micky asked.

Mike, "Everybody is talking about the after party at Duke's after the prom. Man, I have kissed one girl in my entire life and it wasn't Mia! It would be easier to meet up with the fellas. Do you know what I mean?"

Micky isn't surprised. While leaving Mike's house one afternoon, Micky overheard Mike's dad talking. "I know you think I'm hard on you son, but your real father isn't coming back, your mother travels a lot, and I am the only person able to show you what it means to love you." Micky stood at the garage door and ease dropped. He heard Mike's dad say, "No one will ever know, if you don't tell."

They sat on a bench in the park, then Micky said, "Man, you aren't the only guy on the team with mixed feelings. We all go through something. It's noticed, but not spoken. You know, quick glances to avoid direct stares, a gentle touch of shoulders, a bump on the butt while showering (as though celebrating), or the guy who enjoys frequent slaps on the butt. Some people stay straight, others cross over, and some are parallel."

"*Parallel.* That's an interesting use of terms." Mike retorts.

Micky, "You get the point. Ask Mia to the prom. Going on a date does not have to lead to sex. Go and have fun. If the subject comes up, you will know what to say and what to do."

Micky has not dealt with his obsession with Jane. Nor has he been emotionally intimate with anyone else.

Hostility towards his father and feelings of abandonment by his mother fuel rage hidden behind Micky's polite, subtle personality. After informally counseling Mike, Micky realizes he has issues of his own that need to be addressed. What he doesn't know is how to reroute the anger, how to ask for or where to get help. He asked Mike to trust him, but does Micky trust himself? Having not dealt with his own issues, does Micky know how or who he can trust?

———

PAUSE

Try this exercise:

Get a sheet of lined notebook paper. Begin by drawing a line down the center of the paper. Label the left column "Incomplete". Then, use single words to describe unmet feelings, needs, or tasks. For example: apologize, exercise, laundry, forgiveness, anger, etc..... It's your list, continue writing until you want to stop. If you run out of space, flip the sheet of paper over or add sheets of paper.

Label the right column "Complete." Once you work through whatever feelings, needs, or tasks are listed on the left side of your list, move the descriptive 'word' from the left to the right column. Then erase the descriptive word of the completed feelings, needs, or task from the left side of the page.

Once an item on the right side of your completed list is believed resolved, strike through the descriptive word to show that you have let go.

Behaviors tend to recur. Being aware of your feelings and behaviors is important to your

———

becoming. If after you recognize and complete a task, and have stricken that identified item from the list, you later get stuck "doing the same old thing", add the word back to the "Incomplete" column.

Adding a word to the left column of your original list provides a way to challenge yourself to move towards new beginnings. Being aware of unresolved issues is a first step towards healing.

The purposes of this exercise are to be honest with yourself, to openly acknowledge your feelings, and to take actions towards finding a way to work through tough choices. Once you are comfortable with your past, opinions from others is just that... their opinions and perceptions.

Example of a **To Do List**:

Incomplete ------------Complete

Forgive Punch ---------- ~~Punch is forgive~~
Finish painting ----- (   )
(------------) ----- ~~Book is written~~
Back to school --- 3 of 14 classes complete
Keep your list. Time taken to complete unmet

needs (i.e., emotions left unattended) is not as important as making an effort to finish one task before adding to the list. If you do not complete a task on your list, leave the descriptive word on the list. Be yourself and embrace your becoming.

Chapter VI

Move On!

There is no need to explain who you are becoming, nor who you have become. Other people's perceptions of you reflect their expectations for themselves through you. When opinions from others determine who we are, question whose life is being lived.

Sift through information received. Stay grounded! The past is gone. Whatever effects from yesterday, or stuff that prevents you from becoming, hinders your growth...will be in your present until *YOU* learn to package and throw out unnecessary garbage.

What do I mean? We cannot change what has been, but we can embrace today. What wasn't accomplished in the past will not be accomplished today, especially if efforts are made out of malice (an evil attempt at *payback*) – being unprepared.

Abusers and bullies are like a cult; like personalities cling. More often than not, perhaps your instincts have led you away from harm. *Keep going!* Victims can choose to be victimized or victorious!

In the words of my elders, 'A shiny penny becomes dull when exposed to (environmental) elements. Every once in a while, you have to pick it up (the penny) and shine it off. Either way it doesn't lose its value.'

Like yourself! Change what you don't like about yourself and embrace your becoming. Let people's perceptions of who they need you to be, stay with them. Our journey's through life are tough enough without accepting, packaging and carrying someone else's image of who we should become.

1 Corinthians 13:12 (VerseWise) "For now we see through a glass, darkly; but then face to face; now I know in part; but then shall I know even as also as I am Known."

Mini Moment:

School age friends were the best. Sixth through eighth grades (middle school) were especially fun. It was a time of growth and maturation. A time girls clung together being "the girls" and boys clung together being "the boys." Most of us were bused from neighboring counties to attend what was then considered an experimental school, because the District had approved what was known as an "open curriculum."

We were permitted to select seven core courses from a list of classes that had to be completed within three years in order to particulate (graduate) from middle school. Our buildings were named after stars in the solar system (Neptune, Saturn, and Mars). Each building offered course content specific to science, math, and liberal arts.

Students in different grades met for "homeroom" in one of these three buildings. This meant, we gathered each morning, listened to messages, honored our flag and country, then departed to our respective classes. No student was guaranteed to have the same schedule.

We were given a syllabus along with a packet of information that had to be completed before the end of an eight-week session. Two eight-week sessions equaled one semester. Each student was to complete contents within their packet (*this was known as independent learning*), then schedule a test date in the "Test Center".

Tests were not generalized. Each test was specific to the content given in packets. Which meant you studied, learned, passed or failed. If you failed a test, you repeated content in the packet with guidance from an instructor.

Class content was not taught sitting in rows listening to a teacher lecture. We had to read before class and come prepared to discuss whatever might be presented or work in small groups to complete projects. That was an introduction to what is now called, *innovative learning*.

The most important lessons were to think independently, be respective and accepting of others, and never be afraid to challenge the unknown. We weren't expected to know everything, but we were expected to delve deeper into information by reading, to think, and to ask questions.

Education wasn't about going into a classroom to learn from books. Getting an education was about incorporating knowledge researched and published by others, and deciphering what we believed to be important. To decipher information was to pick it apart; to filter what was presented. We were not expected to accept literature as 'truth.' Information published was expected to be tested and retested (aka: Research).

Truth: Every group has a leader. Well in our group, there were many leaders. We all knew too much about life and we were well read. So, when the County decided to introduce us to "Sex Ed" we decided to make active contributions. No touching, much talk, and coming out. Afros, bare chest, mini-skirts, bell bottom pants, and bright teeth were frills to flaunt.

Remember, we were allowed to choose our courses. Once all seats were full classes closed.

———

Once word went out that this class was being offered, a group of us filled spaces to maximize our experiences.

Imagine, teenagers of various ages, races, and grades co-opting to hear what adults felt we should know about our bodies. The joke was kept behind closed doors and we had the last laugh. Let it suffice to say, our teacher understood that we knew what wasn't willing to be taught.

Foundations of our "selves" (plural) begins during the early years. Some believe learning begins within the womb. Others believe socialization is taught by those to whom care is entrusted (e.g., parents, relatives, teachers, friends, etc.).

Behaviors (how a person acts) reflect what a person believes or how a person feels. How one feels about self, situations, or circumstances (real or perceived) becomes that persons reality.

Chapter VII

Then What?!

Dear God, it is me. They tell me I can talk to you. I hope you are listening. They tell me I can trust you and that you are hear for me. They tell me you will never leave me. To me, a kid, that means you will be with me every moment of everyday, wherever I go. So don't leave. I am depending on you to keep your promises.

They have given me this book. It's called a Bible. They say you 'inspired' men to write stories that tell us how we should live. Well, if that is true, as I read this Bible I should learn and live a life guided by you. Don't worry, the Bible given to me is written for kids.

Now let's talk. By the way, how am I to hear your responses to my questions or comments to my concerns?

The child opens the Bible and reads these words, *"My ears had heard of you but now my eyes have seen you"* (Job 42:5 - NIV). *"Ears that hear and eyes that see, the Lord has made them both"* (Proverbs 20:12 - NIV). *"How then shall they*

call on him whom they have not believed? And
how shall they believe in him whom they have not
heard? And how shall they hear without a
preacher?... So then, faith comes by hearing and
hearing by the word of God" (Romans 10:14, 17 -
KJV).

Okay, now I know you can see me and hear
me, and I believe you are with me. My parents
have given me a lamp. It is shaped as an open
Bible with a prayer that reads, "Now I lay me down
to sleep, I pray the Lord my soul to keep. And, if I
die before I wake, I pray the Lord my soul to take."
Why do I have to fall asleep before you take and
keep my soul? If you are with me, why can't you
keep my soul safe now?

The kid opens the Bible and reads, "The fear
of man bringeth a snare: but whoso putteth his
trust in the Lord shall be safe" (Proverbs 29: 25,
KJV), then, "...blessed is the man who fears the
Lord, who finds great delight in his commands...
even in darkness light dawns for the
upright...Surely he will never be shaken, a
righteous man will be remembered forever...his

heart is secure, he will have no fear…" (Psalm
112: 1, 6, 8 - NIV)

Chapter VIII

Continuing...

Mini Moments:

I sit in a room filled with people. None of my friends from daycare or preschool are here. We listen to this lady talk all day. She makes us repeat after her "1, 2, 3, … ', then 'A, B, C,…'. These are numbers and letters. Let us count to 100! Now let us say the alphabet! What is the picture on the card in front of you? Don't say it out loud, write the name of the animal or thing using letters. Why is this important?" Thank God we learned some of this in preschool.

The best part of the day is when we play musical chairs. The next best part of the day is when we go outside onto the playground. There are swings, a sandbox, a teeter totter, a slide, and a thing that you stand on – hold onto bars, then take turns pushing it around in circles. When it is going around fast enough, we jump on, hold onto the bars and ride. It spins and makes us *r-r-really* dizzy.

Second through fourth grades were a breeze.

A solid foundation is easy to build on. Solid meaning 'stable,' as in having a good understanding of what you read. And, knowing what real numbers are. If you don't understand the basics, you will eventually fail. Okay, maybe you won't fail, but you certainly will struggle along the way. So I was taught! *They lied!*

I have to do homework every afternoon. While everybody else is outside playing, I have to do homework. Then, if it is light outside…I can go outside and play. How can I ride to the beach and back before dark, if I have to stay inside and do homework? The answer is, do homework at the beach and be home before my parents, and don't get caught!

That's a plan. Dat and I walk from school and get home by 2 pm. If we cut through the neighborhood, go out sixth street, then through the park, the ride will take about an hour. Homework will already be in our backpacks. We will need water and food. We can be home by 5 or 5:30 pm. Our parents don't get home before 5:45 or 6:00 o'clock.

———

"Hi, I have a plan. Are you interested?" Punch asks.

"No. Your plans always get us in trouble," Dat says.

Punch: "We get in trouble because you tell everything. You have to talk to somebody, anybody. Learn to keep your mouth shut and we won't get in trouble. Are you in or not?"

"What's the plan?" Dat asked.

Punch tells Dat of the plan to ride their bikes to the beach Friday after school. "My Mom will kill me!" says Dat.

"Fine, I'll make better time without you. Stay home," says Punch.

Knowing Dat will tell one of the fellas, Punch decides to alter the plan and go riding another day. If this works, the beach will be a good hide out, a break from his routine. On the other hand, if his parents find out he is riding a bicycle ten miles to the beach, alone, on school days, he is toast!

"Mom, is it okay to go outside and play with Dat after finishing my homework this afternoon?" Punch asked.

"Okay" his Mom says. "I'll be home by 5:30" his Dad interjects.

"Okay" Punch replies. Punch waits until both parents leave for work, then makes sure he has everything in place. His bicycle has air in the tires, a peanut butter and jelly sandwich is ready to go, and a can of Pepsi is on ice. He waits for Dat and Joe so they can walk to school together.

Punch leaves the fellas behind after school. He puts the peanut butter and jelly sandwich in his back pack and cradles the Pepsi in the thermal cup holder on his bicycle. Off he goes! It's 1:45! If he rides fast, he will be at the beach by 2:30.

If I get in the water, will my clothes dry before I get home? What difference does it make if my parents aren't at home? They will know something is off, if they find wet clothes. Hey, that's Bret! What is she doing here? Who is that guy? He looks old. Like an adult. Punch keeps his distance and follows Bret.

Bret and Punch are in the same social studies class. Bret is one year older than Punch, smart, and hangs with an older crowd of eighth and ninth graders. Who is this guy? He has to be in high school or college.

Punch follows Bret up the block before realizing, Bret's and his mom are friends. Bret might tell one of her sisters she saw me today. And, I don't want anyone to know my secret.

Punch rides his bicycle to the south end of the beach. Parks on the sand, lays a towel close the water and begins working on his math assignment. There are ten problems to solve. Punch lays on his back looking up at the clouds. The wind is calm, clouds are drifting north by northeast. He rolls onto his stomach and begins solving math problem number three. After solving problem five, Punch gazes out to sea. The water is light blue and green; Punch can see sail boats and a cargo ship is coming into the port.

The urge to swim is tempting. Punch completes the last of his homework, then strips down to his underwear. He runs into the water and enjoys the warmth of the sea. After swimming free style a few minutes, Punch stops and realizes he is quiet some distance from the shore. As he begins to swim toward the shore, Punch sees Bret and her friend in the water. Punch knows that Bret will see him swim back to shore. There is no way to avoid swimming past them. As Punch approaches, he keeps his head down pretending not to notice them holding one another and kissing. Punch, swims past them, walks onto the shore, dries himself, gets dressed, and throws his backpack onto his bicycle. It is 4:48! He forgets about Bret and heads towards home.

A few days later, Punch passes Bret in the hall at school. "If you don't tell, I won't tell," Bret whispered to Punch.

"Tell what?" Punch asked. Their eyes met; neither said another word.

Punch visits the beach after school at least one day every week. None of his buddies nor his parents know about Punches secret weekly outings. Punch has seen Bret at the beach with that guy, but they pretended to be strangers.

Being near the sea is comforting. Standing along the edge of the sea, Punch pretends that the waves come and go at his will. There is a special connection between Punch and the sea. There have been days when the water has pushed Punch away. Waves have been rough, the temperature of water has been cold, or there are too many sea spurs in the sand that leads down to the shore for him to walk down to the water.

It's Wednesday morning about 0830, "Hey Punch, have you heard?" asks Dat.

"Heard what?" Punch asks Dat.

Dat continues, "You know that girl Bret? She rides the bus from Temple. Well, they found her body near the beach yesterday. Everybody is talking about it! They say her throat was cut and she was raped. Someone found her behind a bar near a bathroom. I'm glad we decided not to ride out to the beach. If there is a killer, that could have been one of us."

Punch listens to Dat without saying a word. His thoughts begin to wonder, 'Is this true? Could that guy have had anything to do with this?'

Out of sight, out of mind. Punch decides it is best to stay away from the beach for a while. Although, he wants to know more. Punch and Bret never openly acknowledged one another while at the beach. 'I hope Bret never told that guy about me. If she didn't want anyone to know she was meeting him in secret, Bret would not have told him, nor anyone,' Punch thought.

Punch sat through class for three days without asking Dat or anyone about Bret. He heard bits of conversations between a few of his classmates about Bret.

Sue: "She was stabbed in the face, neck, and chest."

Moe: "Yeah, I heard she was stabbed over 100 times."

Nip: "Man, who would do that? Who did she piss off?"

Sue: "I heard she was seeing this guy that is in high school. He was questioned by the police last week. The word is, they would skip school and meet at her house or meet off campus."

Nip: "I heard that too. He was going with this girl in the tenth grade and did not want to be seen with someone in middle school."

Dat: "Man, that is messed up!"

Ms. Oveltem, the Dean at Wickem Middle School, spoke over an intercom, "We have a guest. Officer Jones would like to speak with us today about one of your classmates.

Many of you may know that something awful happened to one of your classmates a few weeks ago. Letters were mailed to your parents to inform them of plans for police officers to speak with students."

Officer Jones: "I am Lieutenant Jones, a Detective with the Wickem Sheriff's Department. A few weeks ago, an eighth grade student from your school was found dead near the beach. We are still gathering evidence to figure out what happened. The Sheriff's department and School Board have made grief counselors available on campus in case anyone wants to talk. We are not asking anyone of you to tell these counselors what, if anything, you might know about the deceased or circumstances surrounding her death. The counselors are here because it can be hard for anyone to lose a friend. It can be hard knowing that someone from this school has died.

Even if you did not know Bret, death can be hard for anyone to accept. Please make time and ask your teachers to be excused from class and talk with one of the counselors, if you feel sad, angry, or in any way feel upset about the loss of Bret. Anyone that believes they might know something about Bret that could help us solve her case, please call me at the phone number on this card." Detective Jones walks around in a classroom and hands his business card to each student or lays his business card on their desks. Officer Jones makes an effort to look each student in his or her eyes and asks, "Are there any questions or comments?"

One student asks, "Can you tell us anything about her death?"

Detective Jones: "Bret was 13 years old and in the eighth grade. She was found near the beach here in Wickem. We are looking at video tapes from businesses in the area to see if she met with friends. We do not know if this was Bret's first time at the beach, if she was alone, or how often she may have visited that area. If anyone knows

_____

anything; anything at all about Bret, PLEASE CALL me on my cell phone.

Anyone not in this classroom can stop by the Principal's Office to get my contact information. You can leave a phone number on my cell. You can also call the precinct and leave a message at the office. *I will call you back.* Any information shared will be kept confidential."

Another student asked, "Do our parents need to know if we talk to you?"

Detective Jones: "Anyone with information should probably talk with their parents. But, if you are uncomfortable talking with your parents, please call me and we will work out details together. Remember, the police are gathering information to find out the truth about what happened to one of your classmates."

Detective Jones speaks to Ms. Oveltem privately, then leaves the classroom. A student slips out the back door of the classroom and approaches Detective Jones. "Rumor has it Bret was seeing a guy in high school. He was dating another girl, but I don't know who."

"What is your name?" Detective Jones asks.

"Pearl."

"Pearl, thanks for the tip." Detective Jones smiles towards Sue and walks away. Sue goes to the bathroom, then returns to class.

The following week, Punch and Sue are eating lunch with friends when Punch glimpses Bret's friend in the courtyard. Their eyes meet. Punch pretends not to notice.

The middle and high school campuses are intertwined. The campus Café' is open to students from sixth through twelfth grades. Sue follows Punch's eyes and spots Tim looking at them. "Hey, there is my cousin Tim," she says. Sue waves at Tim and continues talking to Punch.

'Tim?' Punch thinks. 'His name is Tim.' Punch listens to Sue explain how cool it is to have a cousin and brother attend high school at Wickem. Sue tells Punch, "They will graduate in June. Bruce, my brother, could have graduated in December, but he wanted to finish the rest of this year with his friends."

Punch: "And to think, we have another year

before going to high school." Punch is still a bit nervous having seen Tim on campus. He never knew 'his' name and now he wonders what else this 'Tim' might know about him.

Punch and Sue have been friends and run with the same crowd since he was in the sixth grade. Sue talks a lot. Of all the girls in their group, Sue talks more than most. Punch knows better than to say anything to Sue that might call attention to himself. Punch cannot let Sue know that he and Bret shared secrets. Secrets that included Sue's cousin Tim.

Punch had paddled his bicycle to the beach about two weeks after Bret's death. Instead going to the south end of the beach, Punch rode to the park on the North end of the beach. Punch could not remember seeing the guy at beach since Bret's death, although he was nervous that someone might have seen he and Bret together

Occasionally, Bret and Punch would meet across the street from JB's corner street while Bret waited for her friend. They never shared details, but both knew the other did not belong on the beach.

Once, Punch had seen Bret arguing with some guy. Bret was sitting by the water crying silently and the guy was holding her in his arms. After the guy left, Punch rode his bicycle in circles around the block to make sure Bret was alone, then doubled back coming closer so Bret could see him. Punch parked his bicycle across the street in the sand near to shore. Bret walked over and sat in the sand as though sitting alone. "Is everything okay?", Punch asked Bret.

"Yeah", replied Bret. "How much did you hear?"

"Nothing!" Punch exclaimed, making sure to whisper.

"I have to go. I'll see you tomorrow", Bret said.

But the following day, unbeknown to Punch, Bret did not come to school. She had been murdered! Punch could not remember the face of the guy seen holding Bret in his arms. He was not sure if it was 'Tim' or someone else. Tim looked a lot shorter up close. His hair was darker than what Punch remembered, and his shoulders were wide like an athletes'. Then Punch remembered something he had heard Sue telling the gang, "My cousin Tim is training to swim in next year's Olympic games."

Now that Punch knew Tim's name, he imagined seeing Tim all over campus. Punch passed Tim several times a day in the courtyard during lunch, in the library, and while waiting at the bus stop."

"Hey Punch", a voice called. Punch turned around and saw Tim coming closer. "Hey, Sue says you are thinking of joining the junior varsity swim team next year. Coach likes strong swimmers. You will be in eighth grade, right?" Tim asks Punch.

"Yeah. I, uhm… will probably wait and try out in ninth grade", Punch says.

"Yeah, well, I'm a team captain and will be glade to put in word for you. Where do you work out? I haven't seen you swim with the middle school team" Tim says.

"We have a pool at home" Punch replies.

"You should ask Coach if it's okay to practice with the middle school team. Swimming in your backyard is different from swimming in twelve to fifteen feet of water. Unless, your pool at home is that deep?" Tim retorts.

"Naw, it's 4 feet on both ends and 7 feet in the middle. Do you think Coach will let me practice with the team this late in the year?" Punch asks.

"The middle school team practices from 7:30 to 8:15 Monday through Thursday mornings, here - on campus. If you want to practice with them, call me at this number (*Tim writes a phone number on Punch's arm*) and I will pick you on my way to school. You live at 123 Ashmore street, right?" asks Tim.

"Yes. How…" Tim interrupts Punchs' question and says, "Sue told me." Punch has a funny feeling and says, "Okay."

A bus pulls up as Tim walks towards a girl that seems to be waiting for him. "Let me know, Sport" Tim says.

———

Punch gets onto the bus, sits near a window and looks out 'How does Sue know my address? When have Sue and I talked about swimming? Why, after all of these months has Tim chosen now to speak to me?' he thinks. 'What does he want? Why me? Why now?'

At dinner Punch's dad says, "Honey, do you know the young man being questioned in the death of that young girl? Our office has been asked to represent him."

Punch keeps his eyes on dinner as they talk. "No, according to the newspaper he is a senior and honor student at Wickem High. Why?" She asks.

"The girl had information about him in her book bag. There were 'suggestive' pictures of the two of them found in her bedroom. Punch, have you heard anything about this at school? Maybe other kids are talking?" his dad asks.

"People talk. She was in my social studies class", Punch replied.

"Where you friends?" asks Mr. Tate, Punch's dad.

Punch replies, "We didn't talk much. She wasn't one of us. You know what I mean…she had other friends."

"Well, do you know names of her other friends?" his Mom asks.

"Not really", says Punch. "She was stuck up."

"Stuck up? You noticed her, then. When you recall a few names, I'll be here. Trust me kid, I am the only father you have." Mr. Tate takes a bite of out of his chocolate cake, then sips a drink of coffee. "Now this is good!"

How can Punch ask his parents' permission to allow a murder suspect to pick him up, at their home, and drive him to swim practice? They will never, ever, say yes! Unless…

"Mom, Dad" Punch whispers, "Tim has offered to put in a word with Coach Matt, so I can begin training with the middle school swim team. Practice begins at 7:30 Monday through Thursday mornings. If you say it is okay, Tim will pick me up on his way to school. He is captain of the high school varsity swim team."

Mr. Tate hesitates, "Tim who?"

Punch explains, "Tim is my friend Sue's cousin. Sue and I are in home room together; Social studies."

"Does Tim have a last name?" Mr. Tate asks.

"Valesquez. Tim Valesquez" Punch chokes as he talks and eats his chocolate cake.

"Drink your milk or some water" says Mrs. Tate.

Mr. and Mrs. Tate look at one another, then towards Punch. Mr. Tate knows Punch is hiding something. Mrs. Tate opens her mouth to speak and Mr. Tate interrupts, "We will let you know. Why haven't you mentioned joining the swim team before?" asks Mrs. Tate.

"I was going to wait until next year. Thinking maybe you would let me compete in the eighth or ninth grade. Besides, my grades are pretty good, and I haven't been active in school sports. This will prepare me to compete in high school. You both say I am a strong swimmer and should consider being more active in school." Punch takes a deep breath, then continues "Dat and I are thinking about trying out for the swim team next year."

Mr. Tate greets the Valesquez family in his office; "Hello Tim, Mr. and Mrs. Valesquez, please come in. Have a seat. Can my assistant Ms. Riggles get anyone water, a coffee or tea?"

"I would like a cup of tea", says Mrs. Valesquez.

Mr. Valesquez and Tim say, "No."

Mr. Tate begins: "Tim, your principle Ms. Oveltem thought you might need legal representation. The police believe you were involved in the death of a student found near the beach four weeks ago. Have you been questioned by the police?"

Tim replies, "No."

Attorney Tate chimes in, "What was your relationship with Bret Munnings? The eighth grade student from Wickem that was stabbed and left dead near the beach four weeks ago?"

Tim, "We were friends."

Mr. Valesquez interjects, "Tim, Ms. Oveltem called me concerned that the police are investigating you and your relationship with this girl. Son, you need to tell us everything about your friendship with Bret. We need to know how friendly you were with Bret?"

Tim: "We knew a lot of the same people. Bret liked to hang out with us; you know - an older crowd. She was in the eighth grade but dated someone older...that someone was me."

"How far did 'dating' go between the two of you?" asked Attorney Tate. "Did you have sex?"

Tim squirms, looks towards his dad and nods, yes.

Mrs. Valesquez: "Tim, you are 17 years old and that girl was 13! What were you thinking?! Obliviously we need to talk! Are there any other secrets we need to know? Tim, this is serious!"

Mr. Valesquez speaks humbly, "Attorney Tate, it seems we are ignorant of a lot of things. What might we expect?"

Attorney Tate responds, "Tim start from the beginning. I need to know how you met Bret? Start from the beginning...I need details."

Mr. Valesquez: "Perhaps we should schedule another meeting. How much time will you need to spend with Tim and how much will your services cost?"

Attorney Tate: "My daughter Sue is the same age as Bret. They took several courses together. Tim, do you know Sue?"

Tim, "No."

Attorney Tate, "I would like to spend time with Tim to discuss details of his relationship with Bret. Tim let's plan to meet this Saturday. Mr. and Mrs. Valesquez, can I come to your home Saturday around 2 p.m.. I would like to know more before we discuss costs."

Mr. Valesquez: "I need to know what to expect. How much might legal representation cost if Tim is implicated or charged?"

Attorney Tate: "The firm's charges vary. As a Founder and Principle Partner of the Firm, I can afford to spend quality time sorting through preliminary details before discussing money (*Attorney Tate smiles*). Can we agree that I will avail myself to your family this Saturday at 2 p.m.?"

Mrs. Valesquez looks at her husband, then at

Tim and says, "Reputation of your firm is impeccable. Tim hasn't been charged with a crime. He hasn't been implicated in this mess! But, we should be prepared. Thank God, Ms. Oveltem hinted that Tim might be a suspect. Mr. Tate, we await your arrival this Saturday. Can the time of your arrival change to 3 p.m.? I would like for you to meet all of my children."

Attorney Tate responds, "Agreed." He shakes hands with Mr. and Mrs. Valesquez, then with Tim.

Tim looks Attorney Tate in the eyes and asks, "Would it help if I tell you what I know, now?"

Mr. Valesquez interjects, "We have spent over an hour in this office and *NOW* you want to talk? NO! Absolutely, NO Freaking WAY!" Mr. Valesquez hangs his head, runs his hands over his bold head, then apologizes to Attorney Tate, "I am sorry. I sense trouble. We will see you Saturday. By the way, what is your vise?"

Attorney Tate, "I will surprise you. And you, sir?"

Mrs. Valesquez looks at the two men, smiles, then responds, "Saturday at 3 p.m., no surprises."

Once in the car, Tim says to his dad, "I did not kill Bret. She was a friend. Can we just talk about this, the two of you and me? I haven't done anything wrong."

The thirty-minute drive home is quiet. Both of his parents remained silent. Tim sat in the back seat of the car anticipating unknown horrors. He thought, 'What have I gotten myself into? Damn…three years and six months, with four months before I graduate from high school and this happens.'

Then he remembers 'Coach.' If the cops think I had something to do with this mess, I might be disqualified from getting that scholarship! A scandal could ruin my chances of competing in the Olympics! Tim hangs his head in humility, "Lord, whatever happens, please help everyone see that I did not do anything wrong".

They arrive home. The garage door opens. Tim says, "Someone is behind that large brush along the east side of the house. Did anyone see her?"

Mr. Valesquez and Tim get out of the car and walk around the house. They notice a light on in the apartment behind the house. Mr. Valesquez returns to the car and puts the gun from the glove compartment of his car into his pocket. Then he walks around the house opposite of his wife and son. He walks around the pool, goes to the apartment and knocks on the door three times (*knock, knock, knock*).

No one answers. The light inside goes out, there is a sound of ruffling. Mr. Valesquez texts the police notice of an intruder, then signals his wife and Tim to go back.

Mrs. Valesquez and Tim stoop behind the corner of the house just in time to see what appears to be a young girl sneaking out of the back door of the apartment. Tim yells, "Dad, around back! She just went out the back door!"

Mr. Valesquez and Tim followed in pursuit. Thick hedges along the fence provides a shield and the intruder is nowhere to be found.

Two officers came around the house into the back yard and frightened Mrs. Valesquez, who was still crouched in fear. "Mam where is the intruder?"

"My husband and son are behind that apartment. They were chasing someone, I think", retorts Ms. Valesquez. "My husband has a gun in his pocket."

Officer Kelley calls out, "Mr. Valesquez, I am officer Kelley. Officer Jenkins and I have weapons and are coming around to find you. Are you and Tim Okay?"

Tim says, "Yes, we are back here." Both Officers Kelley and Jenkins greet Mr. Valesquez and Tim as they approach the east side of the apartment. The Officer's holster their weapons, "You saw someone back there?"

Tim, "I thought I saw someone in that brush as we drove into the garage. Then we saw a light on in the apartment and heard something break inside."

"We were about to look inside the apartment." Mr. Valesquez extends his hand pointing the way, "After you gentlemen." The Officers, Tim and Mr. Valesquez notice the door ajar and cautiously entered the apartment.

The air smells of roses and brunt paper. Ashes are on the living room table and water is on the floor. A gold goblet appears to have tumbled onto the floor, spilling something red on the sofa and carpet. Pillows and a blanket on the sofa are stained with traces of a moist clear substance. Officer Jenkins dawns gloves and touches the wet spot. "It's not body fluid. Who would have access to this place?"

"My wife uses this apartment as a studio. She paints, enjoys crafts, and writes out here", Mr. Valesquez explains. He continues, "The door isn't locked, so anyone has access to the building."

They here a sound come from the bedroom. Tim offers to investigate as Officer Kelley walks towards the bedroom door. As the bedroom door opens, Tim rushes past Officer Kelley and sees his 14 year old sister Sarah slipping through an outside bathroom door that leads to the patio around the pool.

As Sarah flees, Mrs. Valesquez whispers, "And where are you going?" Sarah stops, turns towards her mother and asks, "Can we do this inside, away from Dad? He is going to have a heart attack and my behind?"

"No. The truth, Now. Who was that and what were you doing?" Mrs. Valesquez asks Sarah.

Mr. Valesquez, Tim, Officers Kelley and Jenkins approach having overheard bits of their conversation. Stone faced, with a smug tone Officer Jenkins turns to Mr. Valesquez and says, "Your wife has found the source of your intruder." Then asks, "Mrs. Valesquez is everything alright?"

Mrs. Valesquez, "Gentlemen, this is our 14 year old daughter, Sarah. This is going be a very long night. Sarah and our son Tim here, have a lot of 'splaining' to do! Please excuse us. Honey we will be in the house."

Mrs. Valesquez, Sarah and Tim begin to walk towards the main house when Sarah and Tim see Bret's sister Kim standing in the shadows. They hope their mother hasn't noticed. Sarah subtly waves for Kim to 'go away.'

Mrs. Valesquez did not notice Kim, but Officer Kelley did! "Hey, you in the shadows, don't move."

Officer Kelley walks towards the person in the shadows, gun holstered with the clip open. "Do not move! Are you armed?" As he approaches the teen, he asks "Who are you and why are you hiding?"

"My name is Kim. Sarah and I are classmates. I wanted to apologize to Kim for getting her in trouble."

"Trouble" asks Officer Kelley. "What kind of trouble?" Mr. Valesquez and Officer Jenkins have joined Kim and Officer Kelley. Sarah, Tim and Mrs. Valesquez continue into the house.

Kim continues, "I wanted to talk with Sarah about something. We were in the apartment talking when we heard her parents come home. We didn't mean to..." Mr. Valesquez interrupts, "Have we met?"

"No Sir. Sarah and I are classmates. I... " Mr. Valesquez interrupts again, "Go home Kim. Now! Go HOME." Officers Kelley and Jenkins chat with Mr. Valesquez then offer to take Kim home.

"It's almost midnight. Attorney Tate will be

here tomorrow. We should sort through this before he arrives. Go to bed Tim and Sarah. This is not over." Mr. Valesquez completes his statement then pours a scotch without offering his wife a drink.

"I am going to bed" says Mrs. Valesquez.

Saturday morning:

Sarah texts Tim 'Lt's tlk.'

Tim's return text 'Cn't'

Sarah 'Mst!'

Mrs. Valesquez has cereal, milk, muffins, and fruit available for breakfast. Tim smells coffee brewing as he comes downstairs. "Hey, what's for breakfast?" he asks his mother. Before Mrs. Valesquez answers, Sarah enters the room, "Mom I am going out. I will be home around noon."

"No one is leaving the house today. Your dad will be down shortly. Tim, Sarah, take a seat at the table. We are having breakfast as a family", Mrs. Valesquez says sternly.

"But Mom, a group of us planned to study this morning. We have a project due Tuesday, and this is the only day the four of us can meet", Sarah replies.

"You will NOT leave this house until this family has met, this day. The two of you do not seem to understand how important the possibility of Tim being implicated in the death of that girl is. Sit! Call your friends, you will have to make other arrangements", Mrs. Valesquez retorted.

Mr. Valesquez enters the kitchen, "Your mother is right. We are a family. Tim, this is serious. Your mother and I need to know about your friendship with this girl. Sarah, you said Kim is Bret's sister? Why was she here last night? What happened outback?"

Tim's cell phone rings. He answers, "Yeah. Uhm. Not now. Later." Tim pulls out the dining room chair next to his mother and begins to sit down. Sarah sat opposite of Tim. Mr. Valesquez stood near the islet as Mrs. Valesquez sat at the head of the table.

"Son, talking about sex with your parents can be embarrassing, but given the circumstances, you need to tell us everything. How did you meet Bret?"

Sarah responds, "Kim and I have been classmates since I was in the sixth grade. Bret use to hang out with Kim and me at their house. They live a few blocks from here. Kim has been upset about Bret's death. She came over last night to talk. Kim says the police plan to talk with everyone that is believed to have befriended Bret. I introduced Tim to Kim and Bret a few years ago." Staring at Sarah, Bret knows his sister is lying.

Tim: "It started with me dating Kim. About two years ago, Kim and I would meet at the beach after school. We didn't know Bret was following us. When Kim found out that Bret knew we were dating, Bret became a brat. We couldn't be alone without Bret threatening to tell their parents. Kim was 14 and not allowed to date."

Mrs. Valesquez interjected "Neither were you! Continue."

Tim continued "Bret saw Kim and I making out on the beach. I told Kim not to worry, I would talk to Bret. The next day, I saw Bret with Sarah at school and asked Bret if we could talk. Bret said 'No,' but later that day we ran into one another during lunch and she told me she would be at the beach after her fifth period class. I knew Kim had gymnastics practice after school, so I drove my bike and met Bret at the beach, so we could talk.

After we talked, Bret agreed not to tell her parents that Kim and I were having sex on the beach. Then Bret kissed me. And, I kissed her back. The next thing I knew, I was making out with Kim's sister." Tim takes a deep breath. Everyone in the room is silent.

"Did you wear a condom?" his father asked wearing a smile.

Mrs. Valesquez cleared her throat while looking at her husband. "Wearing a condom isn't of concern! Tim should not have had sex! With either of them!"

Tim continues to explain "After that day, Bret would come to the beach, wait until Kim left, then tease me. I tried to get Bret to understand that she and I could not have sex again. And that Kim would never understand."

Sarah chimed in "Tim, Kim knows you were close to Bret. I don't think she knows the two of you were, together, like that."

Mr. Valesquez asks, "And you know this HOW?"

"What difference does it make how Kim knew Tim was seeing Bret?" asks Mrs. Valesquez. "This might be the break Tim needs. Is it possible that Kim had something to do with her sister's death?"

The doorbell rang. Sarah answered, "Mom, Dad, Detective Scot is here."

"A Detective, here, now?" Mr. Valesquez asked. "Tim stay in here." Mr. and Mrs. Valesquez go to the door. Mr. Valesquez tells Sarah to 'go into the kitchen.'

Mr. Valesquez greets Detective Scot, "How can we help you?"

Detective Scot: "I am Detective Scot with the Wickem PD. Is there someplace we can talk?"

"Yes, In the den" says Mrs. Valesquez. Mr. and Mrs. Valesquez and Detective Scot go into the den and close the door.

"The two of you probably know that we are investigating the death of Bret Munnings. She was

———
108

an eighth grade student at Wickem Middle school"
Detective Scot says. He continues, "We have
talked with several friends of Bret who think your
son and Bret were close friends. I would like
permission to talk to your son Tim."

Mr. Valesquez says, "Both of our children
knew Bret and her sister Kim. From what our
children have told us there isn't anything unusual
about their friendships with Bret or Kim. Today is
not a good day, our family has plans. Can we
schedule time to meet next week?"

"Me or my partner Detective Kelley, will call
Monday to schedule a meeting with both of you
and your children. Here is my business card. Have
a nice day." Detective Scot smiles and walks past
Mr. and Mrs. Valesquez, then opens the door to
the den and looks around the house while walking
towards the front door. Detective Scot spots Sarah
and Tim standing in the breezeway between the
kitchen and the living room. He waves at the
teens, then leaves.

The family returned to the kitchen, they sat at
the breakfast tablet in silence. Tim and Mr.

Valesquez got up from the table to get a coffee.

Sarah: "Mom, Dad…Kim and I have hung out in the apartment out back after school for a while. A few months ago, Kim came to me upset. There is something going on between Kim and her brother or her Uncle whom she calls dad. She hasn't shared details and I am haven't asked. I think Kim has been molested by her older brother, father or uncle."

Mrs. Valesquez, "Is that what the two of you were talking about last night?"

Sarah, "Sort of. Not having Bret around has been tough on Kim. She says her parents argue more and her brother seems high all the time. Kip, her brother is a senior in Tim's class. Kip plays varsity football. He is expected to get a scholarship to attend college in the fall."

Sarah: "Mom, we snuck out of the apartment because we found your stash of pot, baked cookies and were afraid of getting caught. We were a little high."

Mrs. Valesquez does not respond. Tim laughs out loud then sits down at the table. Mr.

Valesquez clears his throat then asks, "Sarah, why do you think Kim has been molested? What specifically has Kim told you?"

Tim interjects, "I knew Kim was faster than me when we met. She made moves on me that were surprising. As we got closer she told me things. Things about her life. Kim and her brother are a few years older than Bret. When Kim and her brother were younger, they lived in a smaller house and shared a bedroom.

When Bret was old enough to sleep alone, Kip was moved into another part of the house. They have lived in Temple four years.

Kip started hanging with a rough crowd in their old neighborhood. Kip would have Kim run errands for some of his old friends. At first, I thought Kim had dated one of Kip's friends. But when I asked Kim where she had learned some of her moves, she told me that Kip had taught her everything she needed to know."

"What do you mean, son?" asked Mr. Valesquez.

"I asked Kim the same question. Kim said she

and Kip would play house and pretend to baby sit Bret when their parents would go on dates. Sometimes, when their parents were out, Kip would invite his friends over and they would create families. Kip taught Kim how to be a good wife to he and his friends."

"Son are you telling us Kim and her brother…," before Mr. Valesquez could ask the question Tim assures him that "Kim did not say she and her brother, nor his friends had had sex Dad!"

"Then where is this conversation going? And what are you hiding?" Mr. Valesquez asked.

"Kim was not having sex with her brother Kip! Kip was her best friend. Kip protected Kim from their Uncle Charlie. Mrs. Munnings stopped leaving Kip and Kim home alone with their Uncle Charlie after she came home one night and found Uncle Charlie in bed with them naked!" Sarah exclaimed.

Sarah began rambling, "After that Kim and Kip would sometimes baby sit Bret. Kim remembers things their Uncle Charlie, who they refer to as Dad, would do to Kip. She swore to Kip, not to tell anyone! Dad, Mom, you cannot bring this out! Kim, nor Kip would ever hurt Bret.

Bret was the youngest, spoiled, and always snooping around. Bret was a P.I.A! She did the same thing to Kim and me that she did to Tim and Kim. Bret followed Kim and me one day and saw us smoking pot and making out in the apartment out back." Sarah whimpers, "I am sorry Tim. Kim is bisexual. Bret knew our secret and she was going to tell you."

"Sarah, honey" Mrs. Valesquez asks softly, "did you have anything to do with Bret getting hurt?"

Tears begin to trickle from Sarah's eyes. Tim stares at Kim with a blank face as though he doesn't know what to say. "So, you knew Bret and Kim had secrets?" Tim asks Sarah.

"Don't be insensitive and stupid, Tim!" Sarah shouts. "You cheated on Kim by sleeping with Bret and now you want to blame me and Kim!" Sarah gets up from the breakfast table and walks behind the kitchen counter where Mr. Valesquez is standing. Mr. and Mrs. Valesquez watched as

Sarah poured herself a cup of coffee, then returned to her seat in a huff. Everyone in the family knew that Sarah did not drink coffee. As Sarah sipped black coffee, she eyed Tim like a bull ready to charge him!

"Tell the truth Tim. What did you do to Bret? That's really why Kim came over last night. To ask if I knew of your relationship with Bret. Kim suspected you were sleeping with her sister. Everybody knows you are a jock! Everybody knows you have more than your fair share of T T & A! What happened?" Sarah asks in anger.

Tim mutters, "What happened between us was not my fault. Bret came onto me! I don't know how Bret found out about me and Kim. How long she had followed us to the beach. And I don't know why she wanted me. But Bret wanted it! She wanted me bad enough to come onto me. What was I supposed to do? What guy turns down...?"

"Tim, son, you messed up. A lot of guys say no. Especially those of us who know better. Maybe we should have had this talk a long time ago. Didn't you think it strange that a 13 year old girl in middle school would think of having sex with a 17 years old, that is getting ready to graduate from high school?" retorts Mr. Valesquez.

Tim and Sarah were sitting on opposite sides of the breakfast table. It's 10:00 o'clock in the morning and Attorney Tate would arrive at 3:00 o'clock this afternoon. Mrs. Valesquez begins talking, "Cooler heads will prevail. And we have a situation that will involve both of our children. Tim why were you and Kim meeting at the beach? Couldn't you have hung out in school? Who, other than Bret, knew the two of you were meeting at the beach? Was that the only time you and Bret...you know?"

"Mom" Tim hesitates then continues, "I don't know."

Mrs. Valesquez, "Tim I want answers to my questions. If you think my questions are hard to answer, keep these thoughts in your thick skull. A 13 year old girl that you slept with, and whose sister you are known to have dated, is DEAD. The police want to talk with you, and your father and I are about to allow a lawyer into our home to protect YOU. You WILL tell us everything. And, you will answer, honestly, every question posed to you by me, your father, the police, and Attorney Tate. Do you understand?"

Mrs. Valesquez turns to her daughter, "Young lady, I believe you know more than you are telling us. What are you hiding?"

Tim begins, "Like I said, Bret came on to me knowing that I was with Kim. After that happened, Bret continued coming to the beach. She would follow and wait until Kim left, then seek me out. I tried to push her away, but Bret was needy. I didn't have anything to do with killing Bret."

Mr. Valesquez, "What do you mean? What do you know about the death of this girl? Spill IT! Now!"

Tim, "I do not know anything. Nothing! I was as surprised as anyone to hear that Bret had been killed."

Sarah leaves the kitchen. Mrs. Valesquez follows Sarah into the living room. She stands behind Sarah without making a sound. Sarah sends a text to Kim, "What happened btwn the 2 of U?"

Kim texts back "?"

Sarah, "Tell me!' I no U knew"

Kim texts, "So what. It was an accident"

Sarah, "xoxo…need to know!"

Mrs. Valesquez chimed in, "You need to know what? Sarah, talk to me."

Sarah stands from the sofa and turns towards her mother, "Kim knew Bret liked Tim. She suspected they had slept together. Mom, sex isn't like it was; everybody does it."

Mrs. Valesquez, "What do you mean, Sarah? I am not insensitive to emotions of teenagers. Do you understand, someone is *dead?!* It sounds as though you have been a good friend to both Kim and Bret, but now you need to look out for yourself. Please, tell me what you are hiding. I need to know."

Sarah, "Mom, I've told you everything that I know. There were things going on that I don't understand."

Mrs. Valesquez, "Give me your phone."

Sarah, "No!"

Mrs. Valesquez, "Now, Sarah. I want that phone, now." Sarah hands the cell phone to her mother. Mrs. Valesquez read text messages between Kim and Sarah, Sarah and Tim, Sarah and Bret. "You talked with Bret?"

Sarah, "I told you we knew one another."

Mrs. Valesquez, "No, you told us about your relationship with Kim. And, you told us about Tim and Bret sleeping together. You never mentioned talking with Bret. Sarah, how did Bret know to follow Kim to the beach? Why would Bret sleep with an older boy, who was dating her sister?"

Sarah, "You wouldn't understand."

Mrs. Valesquez, "Sarah, you are 14. I don't know what life is like for you. I am concerned that this situation has escalated out of control. Out of control to where you and your brother could face serious consequences. Please...Talk to me. There isn't anything you cannot tell me. I cannot help you if you do not talk to me."

Just as Sarah began to explain, Mr. Valesquez and Tim could be heard arguing in the kitchen.

_____

"Dad, I don't know what happened to Bret! I wasn't there! Besides, I didn't always know when she would show up. The beach was a place for us teens to hang out. A place to escape and play. I was trying to get a part-time job. It wasn't all play."

Mr. Valesquez, "Meeting girls at the beach isn't considered a job! Who else hung out there? Someone saw something."

Tim, "No! There were a few lifeguard positions openings for teens this summer. I applied for a job. We had to show swim competencies to be considered for a job. I knew you would object, so I didn't tell you or mom.

Kim copped out after she failed a timed swim test while fighting the current swimming 100 yards, the week prior to this mess happening. None of our friends would have wanted to hurt Bret. No one knew her! She didn't know, but there was a kid about her age that use to watch us sometimes.

Bret didn't say anything, but I got a feeling they knew one another. I have heard kids around the cafeteria call him Punch. Dad, they were in middle school. What me and Bret did was stupid! I know that! This is wrong. What time is Mr. Tate coming? I need a break. I need to get some air."

Sarah and Mrs. Valesquez joined Tim and Mr. Valesquez in the dining room. Sarah's phone was buzzing with incoming text messages from Kim, 'Cops are here.' 'Cmg ur way.' 'U promised!' 'Call me!' 'Call me! Now!'

Tim grabbed Sarah's phone, read messages texted from Kim and asks, "What did you promise Kim? This is too much. First, I'm stupid enough to sleep with my girlfriend's little sister. Then I learn that my sister is sleeping with my girlfriend. Sarah, tell me if you know anything about Bret and Kim that I ought to know."

Sarah hangs her head, then begins speaking quietly as Tim and her parents listen, "Sit down Tim."

Tim, "Is it that bad? Okay." Tim sits down on a stool at the counter in the kitchen. His dad sat next to Sarah at the dining room table and Mrs. Valesquez stood at the opposite end of the table facing Sarah.

Sarah continued, "It wasn't a mistake. Kim and

I arranged that first date between the two of you; you and Bret. We thought, if Bret messed around with you, it would take the pressure off of us.

Bret caught us petting (*Sarah looked up at her mother, then down at the table*) in the apartment out back. We thought Bret would tell you, so we bribed Bret. Kim told Bret we were experimenting. We assured Bret that you were cool with us, being together and that we would do something special and include her if she would keep a secret.

Kim found out about you and Bret. Kim brushed it off. Kim said that wasn't the first time that Bret had come onto someone she knew. Kim thought the situation that happened years ago between them and their uncle really messed with Bret's head."

Mrs. Valesquez, "That doesn't explain anything. These kids obviously have unresolved issues with intimacy. Is it possible Kim knows who killed her sister?"

Sarah looks into her mother's eyes, "I believe Kim killed Bret."

Tears trickled down Sarah's face. Tim and his

father had perplexed looks on their faces as Mrs. Valesquez spoke, "Why? If these kids are use to sharing sex partners. It wouldn't make since for Kim to kill Bret."

Sarah, "Kim wants to meet me and talk. She is afraid that I will tell Tim that we set him up. I think Kim is still angry about stuff from her past. Not just that one incident with their uncle. Kim's uncle and brother have done some things that she hints of but hasn't shared with me."

Tim sat upright and leaned forward towards Sarah, "Thanks. My prize of a sister has my back! Kim did kill Bret."

The doorbell rang again. Mrs. Valesquez answered the door, "Hi Kim. We were just talking about you."

Kim walked past Mrs. Valesquez intrusively, "Losing my sister is hard. Can I see Sarah, please?"

"We are having company in an hour. Why don't you join us in the dining room? The death of Bret affects all of us. We are all upset" Mrs.

Valesquez extends a hand to show Kim the way into the dining room.

Kim greets Sarah, Tim and Ms. Valesquez then asks if she and Sarah can go somewhere and talk. Everyone in the room looks at Kim and says, "No."

Kim squirms in her seat, hands clasped, arms extended on the table, then says "The police were at our house this morning. I told them you, Tim and I are friends. I told them about Bret and how she liked older boys. Both my sister and I are bisexual. Tim, I know you didn't kill Sarah. A boy from Bret's class has admitted seeing the two of you at the beach together. He told the police that the two of you usually looked happy together. And, my brother has admitted stabbing my sister."

Everyone's eyes are focused on Kim. No one spoke. Sarah stands up, walks over to Kim and hugs her. Sarah whispers into Kim's ear, "Thank God it wasn't you. Forgive me."

Mrs. Valesquez wants to know more but notices the time. The doorbell rings, again. This time Tim answers the door. It is Attorney Tate, "Hi

Mr. Tate. Have you heard? Bret's sister Kim just told us that their brother has admitted to killing Bret."

"No. But we still need to talk. Where are your parents?" asks Attorney Tate.

Tim replies, "They are in the dining room. Come on." Tim escorts Attorney Tate into the dining room where he greets the family and Kim. "You must be Kim? My daughter attended classes with your sister. I am sorry for your loss. What's this I hear about your brother being responsible for Bret's death?"

Kim's voice shivers as she asserts, "My brother told my Mom that Bret was 9 weeks pregnant. She had planned to tell everyone that the baby belonged to him."

Attorney Tate, "Really? When did this conversation take place?"

Kim, "This morning. A Detective was at our house this morning. They spoke with my Mom, then me and Kip. Kip went to the police station to give a statement. My Mom is meeting them at the station."

Kim looks at Sarah, "I really need to talk with you. I have to be home before my mom gets back."

Mrs. Valesquez interrupts, "Your mom left you home alone? You expect us to believe that your mother heard her son admit to killing his sister, then left you home alone while she goes to the police station, knowing her son is about to be arrested for murder?"

Kim "Yes."

Mrs. Valesquez, "Attorney Tate, is there a way to verify this story? Kim you shouldn't be alone at a time like this. You will stay with us until I speak with your mother."

Attorney Tate, 'I will try to contact the Chief of Police.'

The Valesquez family offers Kim something to eat. Kim declines. Tim and Sarah glance sporadically at Kim with questioning eyes. Sarah inches closer to Kim and murmurs, "Kip, really?"

Everyone in the room is fidgety. No one speaks a word. Attorney Tate returns to the room, "Kim, your mother isn't at the local police station.

Who was the police officer, Detective, that came to your home? What was his or her name?"

Kim turns towards Attorney Tate, stares into his face and answers, "Detective Thomas."

Sensing Kim wasn't being completely truthful, Mrs. Valesquez interrupts, "Detective Thomas was one of the Officers at our home that night the two of you were sneaking around out back."

"Yes. He was at our house this morning with another Officer, Detective. They spoke with my mom for a long time. Kip was in his room, but I could hear some of what they discussed. They believed Tim had something to do with Bret's murder. I do not believe Tim would not hurt Bret. Bret had to have things her way. Kip and mom gave Bret everything!

Everything I wanted had to be shared with her! Why Bret? Why not me? Why does everything always center around Bret? She's dead and still everything is about Bret!" Tears begin to slowly drip from Kim's eyes as she continues talking about Bret.

"When we were young, Mom made Kip and I

126

include Bret in everything we did. Everyone loved her. When Bret wasn't the center of attention, she found a way to get attention. I shared Mom with Bret. I shared Dad (Uncle Charlie) with Bret. Kip favored Bret. I was not sharing Tim with Bret!

The little brat didn't think I knew, but I did know. I knew she flirted with Tim. I knew she followed us around town. I knew she spied. And I knew she had to have anything that I wanted. Tim wasn't the first of my friends to sleep with Bret."

Tim and Sarah stared at Kim in amazement. Sarah suspected Kim knew what had happened to Bret. Now Sarah felt convinced that Kim had killed her own sister!

Mrs. Valesquez had inched closer to Kim, placed her around Kim's shoulder lovingly, then whispered "Tell me what happened."

Without looking at Mrs. Valesquez or anyone else in the room Kim said, "I wasn't there. I don't know how it happened. We had a big fight the night before Bret died. Mom and Kip overheard me telling Bret to stop messing around with Tim. Bret said it had happened only once and Kip yelled at me, saying 'it didn't matter anyway.' Kip said we are all too young to make such a big deal out this boyfriend/girlfriend stuff. He said we would both grow out of this fantasy and meet the man of our dreams one day.

I told Bret to find someone her own age and to stop following me around. It gets old. Bret was in the eighth grade!

Tim, I know this seems crazy, but I do not love you. You make me feel special. I like our friendship. I have several friends. Why did you have to have sex with my sister? We were getting along so well."

Mr. Valesquez stepped towards Tim, put his hand over his own lips as though to silence Tim, as Kim continued talking. "Okay, it's out! Tim and I hadn't done anything, but it was wrong for Tim to seduce my sister. Tim did you kill Bret?"

Before Tim could speak Mrs. Valesquez removed her hand from Kim's shoulder, looked at her husband and said, "That's enough. We all need to stop talking."

She turned to Kim and began speaking,

"Young lady, you have admitted having intimate relationships with my daughter, who if you haven't noticed is in this room. And, you have admitted having feelings for my son, who is also in this room. I can't imagine how they feel about you, their relationships with you, one another, or about the death of Bret. I do not believe Tim or Sarah had reason to wish harm on Bret. You are still hiding something."

Attorney Tate had been quiet up until this point, "I came here to hear Tim's version of his relationship with Bret. It sounds as though Kim should speak with her mother and possibly get a lawyer before saying another word."

Kim interrupts, "I don't need a lawyer! I haven't done anything wrong. I need to speak with Sarah, ALONE! That's all I want to do. Sarah, why can't we talk in private?"

Mrs. Valesquez, "We are Sarah's and Tim's parents. Mrs. Valesquez sits in a chair next to Kim, then softly speaks, "My children have to work through their differences. However, there is concern that perhaps Kim believes our children are adults. The world can be a scary place to a child that feels alone. Kim do you feel alone, right now?"

"I am alone. My mom and my brother have been arrested and I don't have anywhere to go. I slipped out the back door and came here to talk with Sarah because I didn't have any place to go," Kim sobs. Sarah walks over and hugs Kim. Tim, Mr. and Mrs. Valesquez look perplexed.

Attorney Tate clears his throat, "Why were your mother and brother arrested? When you arrived, we were told that your mom had gone to the police station. And that Kip had been taken to the police station to give a statement."

Kim whimpers before replying, "None of you understand. There was a time woman married and had babies when they began menstruating. In most girls, menstruation begins long before the age of 13! We aren't little kids.

Okay! Kip, Bret and I did not grow up in a home like yours. We weren't fortunate to have both of our parents around all the time. Your family is not the norm! A lot of single parents raise children alone! A lot of people have problems in their homes. So, what?

My dad left when we were young. My Uncle was a sick s.. of a b..ch! He did things to Kip and me that…weren't natural. My mom has done the best she can to provide us with a good home… to raise us to be normal.   Bret was the youngest. We did our best to protect her, but that wasn't enough. She was too clingy, too needy, too intrusive!

When Mom heard Kip and I arguing, she tried to tame us. She sat us down, listened to me tell my story, then she asked Kip to let it go. But, Kip was mad. Kip knew how cruel Bret could be. He knew that Bret would do anything, I mean anything to get her way. He didn't mean to hurt Bret. Kip was only coming to talk with Tim that day at the beach."

Tim sighs, "Uhm, What? Kip and I did not meet at the beach, that - nor any other day!"

"Let me finish" Kim exclaims, as she wiped tears from her eyes and blew her nose on a tissue. Mrs. and Mr. Valesquez look towards Attorney Tate, "Let her finish" he said.'

Kim rambles, "Kip said he was going to see Tim. Kip said he wanted to find out if Bret was really pregnant or if she was just being a brat – as usual. Kip saw you working your lifeguard post. He noticed Bret talking to some kid at a distance on the beach. When Bret saw Kip coming towards her, she split as though going into the corner store. He caught up with Bret, but she refused to talk with him. Kip said Bret yelled and told him to mind his own business. Kip followed Bret into the alley behind the corner store.

Kip said he grabbed Bret by the arm to stop her and that's when things went south. Bret lashed out at Kip, calling him all kinds of names. She reminded Kip of things that happened when we were young. She even accused Kip of taking advantage of her. I told you, Bret could be fierce!

Kip said Bret pulled out a pocket knife and swung it at him. Kip said Bret blamed him for our uncle raping mom, me, and Kip. She wouldn't shut up! Kip had cuts on his hands from trying to take the knife away from Bret. He lost control."

Attorney Tate interjects, "Did Kip kill Bret?"

Kim, "I don't know. Kip tried to cover up cuts on his hands. When mom came home from work, Bret was still out. Kip and I were having that stupid argument and she asked about Bret. Kip lost it! He called Bret a spoiled little tramp and locked himself in his bedroom.

A few hours later, two officers came to the house. They talked with mom alone and asked that she come to the police station. I knew something awful had happened."

Attorney Tate buts in, "That doesn't tell us your mom and brother were arrested."

"This morning, one of the Detectives said Kip is a primary suspect in Bret's death. I am not sure why mom was taken away", explained Kim.

Attorney Tate continues, "None of this information was expected. Tim, when did you talk with the police?"

Tim responds, "At school. A Detective spoke to our class about a few weeks after Bret died. It wasn't an interrogation, he spoke to everyone, not just me."

Attorney Tate, "What did you tell him? Do you

remember his name?"

Tim responds, "It was Detective Jones. Ms. Oveltem introduced him over the intercom system. After making an announcement about Bret, he asked that anyone who knew her speak with him. I never spoke with Detective Jones alone."

Mrs. Velasquez's soft tone of voice calmed everyone in the room, "I think Kim should stay with us while Attorney Tate finds out what's going on with her family."

Mr. Valesquez listened filled with contempt. He uttered, "These three have kept enough secrets and we still do not know any more now than we knew an hour ago. To recap, my 17 year old son and 14 year old daughter are involved with the same girl, who is now in our home. My wife thinks Kim should stay in our home, while we pay a lawyer to find out what is going on with her brother and mother, who may have been arrested for murder. Although one of our children might be implicated in the murder of Kim's 13 year old sister, who has slept with our son. Does this make sense to you, Shawn (*referring to Attorney Tate*)?"

"It doesn't make sense to me! Hon, I would like to talk with you and Shawn alone. Kids go upstairs. Now. Leave your cell phones on the kitchen table. Kim, that includes you", retorts Ms. Valesquez.

Tim places both hands in his pant pockets, then pulls out his cell phone. Sarah places her phone on the table, as does Tim.

Kim's phone rings, "Mom, where are you?"

Ms. Munnings is silent for a few seconds, then answers Kim, "Kip and I won't be coming home tonight. Where are you?"

Kim answers her mom, "With the Valesquez family." Sarah's parents have invited me to stay with them until you come home. Mom, where are you and Kip?"

Ms. Munnings continues, "Everything will be alright. We will talk later. Please put Mrs. Valesquez on the phone." Kim walks into the kitchen and extends the phone to Mrs. Valesquez. "My mom would like to talk with you."

Mrs. Valesquez accepts the phone and answers, "Hi".

Ms. Munnings, "Thanks for accepting Kim into your home. I can't talk now. It might take a few days to clear up several misunderstandings. Can Kim stay with you until I return home?"

Mrs. Valesquez hesitates, whispers to her husband "Kim might be with us a while, okay?"

He nods in agreement, then Mrs. Valesquez returns to the call, "Sure. We will take care of Kim. Call or stop by when you can." There is a moment of silence between these two women. "By the way, my first name is Sahari", says Ms. Munnings.

Mrs. Valesquez places the phone on the kitchen table and instructs Kim, Sarah, and Tim to "please leave the room."

Attorney Tate begins by saying, "Why don't I leave so the two of you can sort through everything. If I can be a friend, please call me; No charge."

Attorney Shawn Tate is escorted to the door by Bill and Valinda Valesquez. As he leaves, Valinda tells Shawn and her husband "there is something about this family's history that troubles me. Violence and abuse seem to be 'normal' among them."

"This has been a very long day. Should we order out for dinner? Or go out to dinner?" Mr. Valesquez asks his wife.

She responds, "Family decision, let's ask the kids." She then yells upstairs, "Tim, Sarah, Kim – come down here." The three of them stagger downstairs; Sarah, then Tim, then Kim. "Should we go out to dinner or order in?" Everyone agreed - they ordered pizza, chicken wings, and garlic bread sticks - to be delivered.

Early Sunday morning Kim was awakened by the sound of a text message on her phone, "I'm home."

"Okay" she texted back to her mom.

Mrs. Valesquez came into Sarah's bedroom intent on gathering the family for breakfast before church.

Once gathered at the breakfast table, Kim told the Valesquez family that her mother had come home. When asked, Kim did not know where her mother had been, or why Kip was not mentioned during the conversation with her mother.

Kim couldn't stop thinking, "Where had they been? Why didn't mom mention Kip? Has new information been revealed about Bret's death?"

Mr. Valesquez suggested Kim be taken home on their way to church. Sarah asked if she could stay at Kim's house, but her parents insisted it would be best for Kim to spend quality time with her mother.

"Mom, I'm home" Kim shouts as she enters through the garage door. Kim hadn't noticed her mother sitting in a bean bag chair on the floor in the corner of the foyer.

Sahari followed silently behind Kim as they entered the dining room. Ms. Munnings stopped at the entry between the foyer and the kitchen to admire the beauty of her daughter as Kim walked through the foyer, then through the kitchen, and into the living room.

Kim sat in her favorite chair and cocked both feet on the ottoman. She crossed both hands over her head, with her eyes closed. This was the first in several hours that Kim felt relieved.

She was startled when her mother spoke, "You are beautiful. It seems I have not been present with you. Kim, you are my beautiful daughter. I have loved my children without really knowing them."

Sahari sat on the sofa next to the lounge chair, then propped her feet next to Kim's feet before speaking, "Don't leave. Please, sit with me for a while. After a very long and exhausting day, Kip has been sent to stay with your grandparents until he feels ready to come home."

Kim smiles and looks at her mother as though amused. This was the first recollection of grandparents, since, ...well – since before Bret was born! Kip and Kim had spent many days playing around their pound. 'Grandma and Grandpa had cows, hogs, horses, chickens and ducks when we were small,' Kim silently recalled.

"Kim, Kip won't be coming home for a while. I need time to adjust to losing Bret, and Kip choosing to leave home. You have always been the child that did not need consoling. I ask that you be patient, your questions will be answered. I will fill in all of the blanks, but not today. It will take time. I am going to bed," explains Ms. Munnings.

"Mom...Good night" Kim standing behind her mother, kisses Sahari on the cheek, then wraps both arms around her shoulders. "I am staying with you. Good night Mom."

(Pause)

Chapter IX

Interactive Review

The previous story contains a lot of cues to psychological and physical neglect, abuse, bullying, domestic and intimate partner violence. People can get caught up in day to day drama played out in their lives. Cycles of abuse can and do emanate into violence.

Recall cycles of abuse are calm, tension building, eruption of an event (physical, psychological, verbal), then reconciliation (making up). There is no expected order to the cycles of abuse. Abuse, bullying, domestic and intimate partner violence are about "control" or "lack of control." Abusers and bullies lack control. Make time to think through the Mini Moment and answer the following questions:

Is it normal for adults (people 20 and older) to have sexual relationships with children (people 4 through 12 years of age)?

Answer:

_____

_____

_____

_____

_____

_____

_____

During teenage years (ages 13 through 19 is it
normal to experiment by having sex with different
people?

Answer:

_____

_____

_____

_____

_____

_____

_____

At what age is sex socially acceptable?

_____

_____

_____

_____

_____

_____

_____

_____

Hosea 4: 2, 4, 6-7, 10 (VerseWise) reads, "By swearing and lying, and killing, and stealing, and committing adultery, they break out and blood toucheth blood… Yet let no man strive, nor reprove another; for thy people are as they that strive with the priest. …My people are destroyed for lack of knowledge; because thou hast rejected knowledge, I will also reject thee, that thou shalt be no priest to me; seeing thou hast forgotten the law of thy God, I will also forget thy children. As they were increased, so they sinned against me; therefore will I change their glory into shame… For they shall eat, and not have enough; they shall commit whoredom, and shall not increase;

because they have left off to take heed to the Lord."

Hosea 4:14, 16, 18 – 19 (VerseWise) reads, "I will not punish your daughters when they commit whoredom, nor your spouses when they commit adultery; for themselves are separated with whores, and they sacrifice with harlots; therefore the people that doth not understand shall fall…For Israel slideth back as a backsliding heifer; now the Lord will feed them as a lamb in a large place…Their drink is sour; they have committed whoredom continually; her rulers with shame do love, Give ye. The wind hath bound her up in her wings, and they shall be ashamed because of their sacrifices."

Chapter X

Present...

Mini Moments:

I know you're still with me and you listen. Too many things have happened or gone past me, and I have wanted many times to dismiss you. But every time I try to ignore your presence, not wanting to believe anything bad would happen because you are with me, you show me how things I believe are painful and blessings. How you make decisions are not for me to understand. I don't expect an answer, but it is only fair to tell you that I know you are keeping your promises.

The Bible given to me as a child is at home, but don't worry there are Bible's everywhere I go. In churches, in schools, and at work. I have even been given another Bible.

So many people share something called 'trust' in you. People, who like me, cannot see you but know you are real. The hard part of talking with you is not believing you exist, it's not seeing you. It is feeling a little strange knowing that someone was born into the flesh, singled out, treated horribly, then murdered. After dying a physical death, stories in the Bible say your spirit left the flesh, went back to your father in heaven, then appeared to humans again, just to show us that you love us and are still with us. The Bible calls this the 'resurrection'.

According to the book, people that trust and believe you exist and resurrected have a good chance of being like you: Forgiven of things we do wrong and being born again after death.

John 11: 17, 19 – 27 (KJV) reads, "Then when Jesus came, he found that he had lain in the grave four days already...many of the Jews came to Martha and Mary to comfort them concerning their brother. Then Martha, as soon as she heard that Jesus was coming, went and met him: but Mary sat still in the house. Then said Martha unto Jesus, Lord, if thou hadst been here, my brother had not died. But I know that even now, whatsoever thou wilt ask of God, God will give it to thee. Jesus saith unto her, Thy brother shall rise again. Martha said unto him, I know that he shall rise again in the resurrection at the last day. Jesus said unto her, I am the resurrection and the life, he that believeth in me, though he were dead, yet shall he live. And whomsoever liveth and believeth in me shall never die. Believest thou this? She saith unto him, Yea, Lord: I believe that thou art the Christ, the Son of God, which should come into the world."

1980's - What's up? This journey hasn't gotten easier! How many pits must I fall into before peeping at a little light? Have I mentioned these pits have caves? Deep caves!! Maybe you expect a little independence crawling out of these pits. Yes, I know I have not loved you with my whole heart: I have strayed and not sought your guidance. I am asking for help now. Will you meet me along the way? I'm not feeling your presence. Yeah, I know. You are here, somewhere. They told me I'm not to question you. I am not to do anything that will insult you. Well, I don't believe them. I believe you want me to keep being honest with you. I believe you created me to not only trust you, you expect me to trust, to be obedient, and to have patience. Well, I have no patience, I am too honest, and I am trying to trust you! Yes, I have tried trusting people. No that hasn't worked in my favor. Just like trusting you is hard and often disappointing. No, I will NOT QUIT!! I will keep talking to you. Maybe one day you will help me understand your purposes for leaving me in the pits of these valleys. By the way, it's cold, it feels lonesome, and it's dark (even when the sun shines), and I don't like your choices. There! I have said my peace. NO, I am not at peace. AMEN!

Job complained with bitterness in chapter 23: 2 - 17 (NIV)... *Even today my complaint is bitter; his hand is heavy in spite of my groaning. If only I knew where to find him; If only I could go to his dwelling! I would state my case before him and fill my mouth with arguments. I would find out what he would answer me, and consider what he would say. Would he oppose me with great power? No, he would not press charges against me. There an upright man could present his case before him, and I would be delivered forever from my judge. But if I go to the east, he is not there; if I go to the west, I do not find him. When he is at work in the north, I do not see him; when he turns to the south, I catch no glimpse of him. But he knows the way that I take; when he has tested me, I will come forth as gold. My feet have closely followed his steps; I have kept to his way without turning aside. I have not departed from the commands of his lips; I have treasured the words of his mouth more than my daily bread. But he stands alone, and who can oppose him? He does whatever he pleases. He carries out his decree against me, and many such plans he still has in store. That is why I am terrified before him; when I think of all this, I fear him. God has made my heart faint; the almighty has terrified me. Yet I am not silenced by the darkness, by the thick darkness that covers my face.”*

Chapter XI

Continued...

Four days pass, Kim Munnings sits in her bedroom remembering events from the past few months. Her sister Bret is dead, her brother Kip has moved out, her mother has not offered explanations and Kim is manic trying to bury her own feelings. When will Sahari Munnings be ready to talk? And who killed Bret? Why? Whatever she doesn't know is not going to stop Kim from delving deeper. Tim would not hurt anyone. Bret had forced herself on Tim for weeks. That little brat had secrets! Lots of secrets.

Kim and Sarah's friendship has been distant. They talked via text messages and video chats. If she could not meet and work things out with Sarah, how would Kim survive. 'Sarah is my best friend' Kim thinks. 'Why is everyone keeping secrets?'

Sarah's parents forbid the girls from seeing one another. At school, Sarah avoided Kim. Sarah being in 8th grade, although very robust in stature and Kim, a first year student in high school

(9th grade) didn't help their situation.

Both middle and high school classes share the same campus. Before everything happened, Kim and Sarah would arrange to share lunch. Maybe setting Bret up as a lure for Tim was a bad idea. The girls really believed Bret could be a distraction by flirting with Tim. Never in a million years had they dreamed of Tim and Bret sleeping together.

"Kim" Sahari calls out to her daughter, "don't make plans after school this afternoon. I need you home by 3 o'clock - Okay?"

"No. I already have plans," Kim retorts.

"Not today. Do not detour, come straight home after school today. I will be home by 3:30!" Sahari shouts.

Sahari waits for Kim to leave then sends a text message to Kip, "Hi – Hv U forgiven me?" She waits a few minutes then gets into the shower.

Feelings of shame, guilt and doubt fill Sahari's emotions as she showers, 'I should have done this a long time ago. I promised to protect my children. I promised they would not suffer because of our past, my past. How can I tell them the truth? How do I explain that their father is alive? They might not understand, but I owe them an explanation. I owe them…they need to know everything."

As she dries her body, then gets dressed. Sahari prepares to take a trip and visit Kip. She texts Kim, 'Chg of plns. Will be hm by 8 pm.'

Soft jeans and a T-shirt will be comfortable for the drive. She pulls her hair back, then up into a pony tail, then wraps a scarf around her head. No make-up and post earrings to brighten my face. This isn't a pleasure trip.

As Sahari approached her parents farm, her face tightened, and a tear falls from one eye. She sniffs and dries her right eye. She thinks, 'I haven't been home in almost 13 years.

An array of emotions came rushing upon Sahari as she turned onto the property. She stops the car and opens the door. As she steps onto the black soil that paves an old dirt road, Sahari closes her eyes, feels rays from the sun upon her face, and smells the scent of freshly cut grass mixed with clear air. A breeze of wind blows into her face. Sahari is home.

She was delivered by a midwife in the old house that sits on the hill. Her family has owned and lived on this land for over 100 years. Family members told stories of how Sahari and siblings brought life into their parents' lives. Sapodilla trees align the drive way. Pecan trees, azaleas, citrus trees are scattered throughout the property surrounding her parent's home.

Sahari learned how to milk cows, gather chicken eggs, roll bales of hay, and groom horses as a child. This farm was a place of solace, with hidden fears. Early childhood memories had become obscured by repeated tragedies, kept silent to protect 'the family's name and reputation.'

As Sahari exited her car two dogs greeted her with barks and wagging tails, followed by a thin female about 5 feet 6 inches tall. Before Sahari and her mother embraced, she heard a man's voice, "What brought the kid home?" As the man approached Sahari quickly headed in his direction "Dad?"

Her mother smiled, stood back, and waited as Sahari hugged her father. After a few minutes,

Sahari's mom, standing within inches of the father and daughter, hugged her daughter with tears streaming from both eyes. Sahari was overwhelmed with feelings of comfort and joy. She was so overcome with emotions that she did not see Kip standing on the porch watching.

Kip waved towards his mother, then went back into the house. Sahari and her parents walked around the acreages of land that surround the house. There was small talk of plants, the weather, farm animals that Sahari once considered as pets. They reminisced about of the past until Sahari recalled an event that was not pleasant. Instead of bringing up the past, she withheld her thoughts and feelings, then changed the conversation.

Sahari knew what needed to be done. As unpleasant as the past had been, many of her past experiences had unknowing and adversely affected the lives of her children. Unresolved feelings silenced by fear of the unknown needed to come out. Her children deserved to be free of her guilt. Sahari also knew that she nor her children were directly responsible for the death of her daughter Brett. Something she nor her parents had mentioned.

"Hi Kip" Sahari says softly as she greets her son. Kip had retreated to his bedroom as an attempt to delay seeing his mother. He sat on his bed quietly with head phones on listening to music. Kip knew Sahari had entered the room. He had also heard her speak to him. Kip did not look at his mother. He ignored Sahari's presence by turning his body towards the window.

Sahari walked around Kip and stood between the bed and the window to block his view. Kip stared at his mother with a blank face. "I am not coming back. Not now. Please leave." Kip spoke soft and stern to Sahari.

"I am not her to ask you to come home. Nor am I here to stay. Kip, sometimes people can't meet our needs. There are many things that have shaped my life that have in many ways spilled over to my children. As I drove here, there were so many things I wanted to tell you. I felt you were due explanations for things happening that were beyond your control."

Sahari smiles, then sits on the bed next to her son. "Being here, I know that my past was built on a solid foundation. I know that circumstances and situations helped build character within me. I hope a little of what my parents shared with me spills into you.

You are not responsible for Bret, nor Kim. The three of you are my children. My children are my responsibility. Bret was my responsibility.

The last time I saw my parents, I was carrying Bret. They would have done anything to convince me to stay and give birth on this farm. But I wanted to leave. I felt a need to live my life with a sense of independence.

Bret was young, but I could see that free spirit in her eyes. Bret's death was not an accident, but the person that killed Bret is responsible for her death. We may never know who violated our family by snatching Bret away from us. And I am saddened that so many people blamed you. You did everything humanly possible to save her. If you had not gone looking for Bret and seen her

laying on the ground, she would have died alone."
Kip's eyes became watery, but he refused to cry.
At seventeen, Kip expressed a hardness of heart
and he was determined to remain behind that wall
of silence.

Sahari sat close to her son and placed an arm
across his shoulder, "Sometimes people take
power and sometimes power is given. You will
learn to distinguish when you have power to give,
power to share, as well as when and which forms
of power to take. Never allow anyone to silence
you. Bullies need buddies. Silence gives bullies
the false belief that they are in control."

She stood and began pacing, "Take control of
your life by talking about things that make you
uncomfortable. Do not give this murderer power
by being angry. Take away his or her power by
being confident in what you know. And only you
know what happened the day you found Bret."

Sahari kneels beside the bed next to Kip,
"They should have verified all of the facts. Your
father served this country with most of those
people in law enforcement. Their errors in

judgement and shear willingness to accept at face value that you would murder your sister was wrong. I promise you Kip, the truth will prevail."

Sahari stood and faced the window with tears trickling from both eyes. After gaining her composure, Sahari wiped her face and put on a smile. She opened the Bible that was laying on Kip's pillow, then said, "Who you know is not as important as what you know and how you use that information. Son, I am glad to see that you know to whom you can turn and who to truly trust."

Sahari read to Kip from the book of Judith 2: 2-5, 10 -13 (VerseWise), *"So he called unto him all of his officers, and all of his nobles, and communicated with them his secret counsel, and concluded the afflicting of the whole earth out of his own mouth. Then they decreed to destroy all flesh that did not obey the commandments of his mouth. And when he had ended his counsel, Nabuchodonosor king of the Assyrians called Holofernes the chief captain of his army, which was next unto him, and said unto him; This saith the great king, the lord of the whole earth, Behold,*

*thou shalt go forth from my presence, and take
with thee men that trust in their own strength, of
footmen and hundred and twenty thousand; and
the number of horses with their riders twelve
thousand… Thou therefore shalt go forth and take
beforehand for me all of their coasts; and if they
will yield themselves unto thee, thou shalt reserve
them for me until the day of their punishment. But
concerning them that rebel, let not thine eye spare
them; but put them to the slaughter, and spoil
them wheresoever thou goest. For as I live, and by
the power of my kingdom, whatsoever I have
spoken, that will I do by mine hand. And take thou
heed that thou transgress none of the
commandments of thy lord, but accomplish them
fully, as I have commanded thee, and deter not to
do them.'*

Sahari then turns back to her son, "I have to
go, Kip. Know that I love you. Know that this too
shall pass. Know that Bret will always have a
place in our hearts. And know that it is okay to
allow yourself to feel and show to emotions. If you

won't talk to me, talk to my parents (*Sahari smirks*). Talk when you feel compelled to talk and feel free to tell the truth. It takes work, a conscious effort, to open up to others and not keep your feelings bottled up inside of you." Sahari leans forward and hugs Kip.

Kip squares face to face with Sahari, looks directly into her eyes then asks "Mom, when will you come back?" Sahari replies, "Soon. And maybe Kim will come with me.'

Chapter XII

Awakening...

As Sahari drove back to Wickem thoughts of her childhood emerged. She prayed that her son Kip could find peace within himself. Kip had done everything possible to save Bret. He had tried to protect Bret from everything. But no one could have protected Bret - *from Bret!*

Kip and Kim had practically raised Bret, since Sahari was a single parent who had worked eight to twelve hour nights. These kids had been child parents to their infant sister.

Sahari knew Kip had secrets. She vaguely recalled things the children had tried to tell her years ago. Could PJs brother really have harmed them? Had she been remiss by dismissing their cries for help.

Without a father role model, Kip had assumed roles of 'a man' by watching his Uncle and television. The same Uncle that had coached Kip and Kim to sleep in her bed naked while she worked nights.

Bret had a free spirit. Dead at the age of 13,

Bret had experienced life more than many adults.

Circumstances surrounding Bret's death had not been told to Kip, nor to Kim. Sahari had tried to protect her children. She had not told them truths about their father. Sahari had minimized or avoided conversations about PJ Manning.

Before Bret was born PJ and Sahari's relationship had changed dramatically! Sahari and PJ had to do what was best for their family.

Raised on a farm, Sahari had learned the beauty of quietness, stillness of the earth, and peace that comes with community. Their families had been friends long before PJ or Sahari were born. Sahari and PJ had been friends since childhood.

Sahari wanted and believed she should tell PJ about Bret. Bret was born, named, and died not knowing her father. Sahari realized that PJ does not know Bret!

Keeping secrets was something else Sahari had mastered. As a child, Sahari learned that 'girls are to be seen and not heard.' Sahari's quaintness remained reflective of a culture with which she is all too familiar.

Sahari felt she had loss Kip, their first born child to depression. She felt distant from Kim, their second child. And, she had recently buried Bret, their youngest child – the baby. She had been estranged from her husband for almost fourteen years!

Once back in Wickem, Sahari called Kim. Kim's phone rang, but there was no answer. Sahari left a message, "Be home when I get there. I'll be home within 15 to 20 minutes."

As Sahari pulled into the drive way, she sighed and made a mental list of things to be done. Kim should be taken to see her grandparents and Kip needed time to accept that the loss of Bret was not his fault.

Getting in touch with PJ would be a daunting task. A task that required candor and diplomacy befitting of a lady. It was time to reunite with PJ, silently – in secret.

Sahari sat in the car and allowed herself to feel pain, as well as sadness. There had not been time to grieve her losses. She prayed, then opened the bible on her phone and read from the book of Isaiah 47: 8-9 (VerseWise, KJV), *"Therefore hear now this, thou that art given to pleasures, that dwellest carelessly, that sayest in thine heart, I am, and none else beside me; I shall not sit as a widow, neither shall I know the loss of children. But these two things shall come to thee in a moment in one day, the loss of children, and widowhood; they shall come upon thee in their perfection for the multitude of thy sorceries, and for the great abundance of thine enchantments."*

———————

Notes from the Author

Our live journeys are mimicked by no other. Some behaviors are learned while other behaviors develop as responses to stimuli. What has shaped your behaviors? Looking into lives of others is easy. Open and honest introspections (looking inside your own life) might not be as easy. A certain, freedom, comes with self-introspection and willingness to share.

Mimi moments (short stories) written in scenarios, along with short task in PEEPED are intended to evoke thoughts on healthy and unhealthy behaviors. Abuse, bullying, domestic and intimate partner violence should not be kept secret. Such abnormal behaviors diminish when exposed. **Abuse, bullying, domestic and intimate partner Violence are everybody's business!!**

Characters in PEEPED are not real. Content and definitions are real.

We can easily get caught up in 'the stories' or events that happen in our lives. Once we look past the initial 'awe' of what was, or what has happened, and realize the blessings that follow an event, somehow the stories become less significant. Our blessing can be found within lessons learned.

Everybody needs something in which they can believe. That something for me is grounded in blind, as well as biblical faith. Life does not come with 'one size fits all' instructions, text, or guidance. Challenge yourself to look beyond where you have been and seize moments of each day, then just be - you.

Scriptures quoted throughout PEEPED are from:

1. VerseWise Bible, KJV for iPhones (2018, 2017), VDUB Software, LLC. VerseWise offers biblical readers access to the Deuterocanon, also known as the lost books or apocrypha.

2. Scripture quotations marked (NIV) are taken from the Holy Bible, New International Version®, NIV®. Copyright © 1973, 1978, 1984, 2011 by Biblica, Inc.™ Used by permission of Zondervan.

3. King James Version (Free download) for
iPhones; Tecarta, Zendesk.

NATIONAL CRISIS ORGANIZATIONS AND ASSISTANCE RESOURCES:

The National Domestic Violence Hotline
    1-800-799-7233 (SAFE)
    www.ndvh.org

National Dating Abuse Helpline
    1-866-331-9474
    www.loveisrespect.org

Americans Overseas Domestic Violence Crisis
    Center
    International Toll-Free (24/7)
    1-866-USWOMEN (879-6636)
    www.866uswomen.org

National Child Abuse Hotline/Childhelp
    1-800-4-A-CHILD (1-800-422-4453)
    www.childhelp.org

National Sexual Assault Hotline
    1-800-656-4673 (HOPE)
    www.rainn.org

National Suicide Prevention Lifeline
    1-800-273-8255 (TALK)
    www.suicidepreventionlifeline.org

National Center for Victims of Crime
    1-202-467-8700
    www.victimsofcrime.org

National Human Trafficking Resource
    Center/Polaris Project

Call: 1-888-373-7888 | Text: HELP to BeFree
(233733) **www.polarisproject.org**

National Network for Immigrant and Refugee
Rights
1-510-465-1984
www.nnirr.org

National Coalition for the Homeless
1-202-737-6444
www.nationalhomeless.org

National Resource Center on Domestic Violence
1-800-537-2238
www.nrcdv.org and **www.vawnet.org**

Futures Without Violence: The National Health
Resource Center on Domestic Violence
1-888-792-2873
www.futureswithoutviolence.org

National Center on Domestic Violence, Trauma &
Mental Health
1-312-726-7020 ext. 2011
www.nationalcenterdvtraumamh.org

CHILDREN
Child-help USA/National Child Abuse Hotline
1-800-422-4453
www.childhelpusa.org

Children's Defense Fund
202-628-8787
www.childrensdefense.org

Child Welfare League of America
    202-638-2952
    www.cwla.org

National Council on Juvenile and Family Court
    Judges: Child Protection and
    Custody/Resource Center on Domestic
    Violence
    1-800-527-3233
    www.ncjfcj.org

Center for Judicial Excellence
    www.centerforjudicialexcellence.org

TEENS
Love is respect
    Hotline: 1-866-331-9474
    www.loveisrespect.org

Break the Cycle
    202-824-0707
    www.breakthecycle.org

Domestic Violence Initiative
    (303) 839-5510/ (877) 839-5510
    www.dviforwomen.org

Deaf Abused Women's Network (DAWN)
    VP: 202-559-5366
    www.deafdawn.org

Women of Color Network
    1-800-537-2238
    www.wocninc.org

_____

INCITE! Women of Color Against Violence
www.incite-national.org

LATINA/LATINO
Alianza
    1-505-753-3334
    www.dvalianza.org

Casa de Esperanza
    Linea de crisis 24-horas/24-hour crisis line
    1-651-772-1611
    www.casadeesperanza.org

National Latin@ Network for Healthy Families and
    Communities
    1-651-646-5553
    www.nationallatinonetwork.org

IMMIGRANTS
The National Immigrant Women's Advocacy
    Project
    (202) 274-4457
    http://www.niwap.org/

INDIGENOUS WOMEN
National Indigenous Women's Resource Center
    855-649-7299
    www.niwrc.org

Indigenous Women's Network
    1-512-258-3880
    www.indigenouswomen.org

ASIAN/PACIFIC ISLANDERS
Asian and Pacific Islander Institute on Domestic

Violence
1-415-954-9988
www.apiidv.org

Committee Against Anti-Asian Violence (CAAAV)
1-212- 473-6485
www.caaav.org

Manavi
1-732-435-1414
www.manavi.org

AFRICAN-AMERICANS
Institute on Domestic Violence in the African
American Community
1-877-643-8222
www.dvinstitute.org

The Black Church and Domestic Violence
Institute
1-770-909-0715
www.bcdvi.org

LESBIAN, BI-SEXUAL, GAY, TRANSGENDER,
GENDER NON-CONFORMING
The Audre Lorde Project
1-178-596-0342
www.alp.org

LAMBDA GLBT Community Services
1-206-350-4283
**http://www.qrd.org/qrd/www/orgs/avproject
/main.htm**

National Coalition of Anti-Violence Programs

1-212-714-1184
www.ncavp.org

National Gay and Lesbian Task Force
1-202-393-5177
www.ngltf.org

Northwest Network of Bisexual, Trans, Lesbian &
Gay Survivors of Abuse
1-206-568-7777
www.nwnetwork.org

Trans Lifeline
877-565-8860
www.translifeline.org

ABUSE IN LATER LIFE
National Clearinghouse on Abuse in Later Life
1-608-255-0539
www.ncall.us

National Center for Elder Abuse
1-855-500-3537
www.aginginplace.org

MEN
National Organization for Men Against Sexism
(NOMAS)
1-720-466-3882
www.nomas.org

A Call to Men
1-917-922-6738
www.acalltomen.org

Men Can Stop Rape
1-202-265-6530
www.mencanstoprape.org

Men Stopping Violence
1-866-717-9317
www.menstoppingviolence.org

American Bar Association Commission on
Domestic Violence
1-202-662-1000
www.abanet.org/domviol

Battered Women's Justice Project
1-800-903-0111
www.bwjp.org

Legal Momentum
1-212-925-6635
www.legalmomentum.org

Womenslaw.org
www.womenslaw.org

National Clearinghouse for the Defense of
Battered Women
1-800-903-0111 x 3
www.ncdbw.org

Legal Network for Gender Equity
nwlc.org/join-the-legal-network/

Other Authored Works...

Living Beyond Survival: Laughing, Loving,

Sharing...Life! By Van Johns (2011).
AuthorHouse Publishing.

Paths to Empanelment (Accepted, April 3, 2018).
Journal of the American Academy of Nurse
Practitioners.

Ray's theory of bureaucratic caring: A conceptual
framework for APRN Primary Care Providers
(2015). International Journal for Human
Caring, 19 (2).

Made in the USA
Lexington, KY
22 September 2018